Evaluating health promotion
Practice and methods

THIRD EDITION

Edited by

Margaret Thorogood and

Yolande Coombes

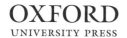

OXFORD
UNIVERSITY PRESS

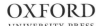

OXFORD
UNIVERSITY PRESS

Great Clarendon Street, Oxford OX2 6DP

Oxford University Press is a department of the University of Oxford.
It furthers the University's objective of excellence in research, scholarship,
and education by publishing worldwide in

Oxford New York

Auckland Cape Town Dar es Salaam Hong Kong Karachi
Kuala Lumpur Madrid Melbourne Mexico City Nairobi
New Delhi Shanghai Taipei Toronto

With offices in

Argentina Austria Brazil Chile Czech Republic France Greece
Guatemala Hungary Italy Japan Poland Portugal Singapore
South Korea Switzerland Thailand Turkey Ukraine Vietnam

Oxford is a registered trade mark of Oxford University Press
in the UK and in certain other countries

Published in the United States
by Oxford University Press Inc., New York

© Oxford University Press, 2010

British Library Cataloguing in Publication Data

Data available

Library of Congress Cataloging in Publication Data

Evaluating health promotion: practice and methods / edited by Margaret Thorogood and Yolande
Coombes. — 3rd ed.
    p. ; cm.
  Includes bibliographical references and index.
  ISBN 978-0-19-956929-8 (alk. paper)
  1. Health promotion—Evaluation. I. Thorogood, Margaret. II. Coombes, Yolande.
  [DNLM: 1. Health Promotion—standards. 2. Outcome and Process Assessment (Health
Care)—methods. 3. Program Evaluation—methods. WA 590 E915 2010]
  RA427.8.E95 2010
  362.1—dc22   2010010912

Typeset in Minion by Glyph International, Banglore, India
Printed in Great Britain by the MPG Books Group, Bodmin and King's Lynn

ISBN 978–0–19–956929–8

10 9 8 7 6 5 4 3 2 1

Contents

List of contributors

Virginia Berridge
Professor of History,
Centre for History in Public
Health,
London School of Hygiene and
Tropical Medicine,
London, UK

Annie Britton
Senior Lecturer in
Epidemiology,
Division of Population Health,
University College London,
London, UK

Steven Chapman
Chief Technical Officer,
Population Services
International,
Washington DC, USA

Yolande Coombes
Consultant,
Water and Sanitation Program,
World Bank,
Nairobi, Kenya

Jane Cowl
Programme Manager,
Patient & Public Involvement
Programme,
National Institute for Health
and Clinical Excellence, UK

David Ellard
Senior Research Fellow,
Warwick Medical School,
University of Warwick, UK

Melvyn Hillsdon
Associate Professor of Exercise
and Health Behaviour,
School of Sport and Health
Sciences,
University of Exeter, UK

Rachel Jewkes
Director,
Gender and Health Research
Unit,
Medical Research Council,
Pretoria, South Africa

Dalya Marks
Lecturer,
Department of Public Health
and Policy,
London School of Hygiene and
Tropical Medicine
London, UK

Suzanne Parsons
Senior Research Associate,
Picker Institute Europe,
Oxford, UK

John Powell
Associate Clinical Professor in
Epidemiology & Public Health,
Warwick Medical School,
University of Warwick, UK

Warren Stevens
Health Policy Advisor,
Population Services
International,
Washington DC, USA

Carol Tannahill
Director,
Glasgow Centre for Population
Health,
Glasgow, UK

Margaret Thorogood
Professor of Epidemiology,
Warwick Medical School,
University of Warwick, UK

Part I

Overview

Chapter 1

Introduction

Yolande Coombes and
Margaret Thorogood

Writing the Introduction to the first edition of this book a decade ago, our focus was on the need to establish a credible evidence base for health promotion through rigorous quantitative and qualitative evaluation studies, and one of our concerns was to move on from the sterile argument over superiority between quantitative and qualitative methodologies. At that time, health promotion evaluation was still an emerging discipline, borrowing extensively from the social sciences, but without a clear methodological position. Four years later, by the time of the second edition, health promotion evaluation had a clearer focus, embracing both quantitative and qualitative methods, although not always explicitly. However, the evidence for efficacy and effectiveness of health promotion initiatives remained patchy and one of the key themes in that edition was the need for further strengthening of the evidence base.

We ended the second edition with a call for more tolerance across disciplinary boundaries and greater integration of approaches, arguing that 'no one approach should be considered the exclusive domain of one group of researchers'. Since then, 'mixed-methods' research has become a mainstream academic activity with its own journal and conferences. The debate over method choice is over. Moreover, the need to develop and evaluate complex interventions (and health promotion interventions are almost always complex) using a mixed-methods approach is now an accepted view (Craig *et al.* 2008) but, despite this, using a mixed-methods approach to evaluation remains uncommon (Lewin *et al.* 2009). O'Cathain *et al.* (2008) have argued that it is crucial that we make more of mixed methods in health research. Similarly Pope and Mays (2009) report that qualitative research tends to take a supportive role, and is rarely fully integrated with quantitative methods. They ask 'What happened to the idea that we could learn more from the fact that qualitative research looks at things in a different way?' They argue that the creative tension between methods can be positive and that different and sometimes opposing insights gained from different methods can tell us something new (Pope and Mays 2009). The trend in health promotion is to emphasize impact and outcomes in evaluation and less attention is given to process and context in the construction of the health promotion evidence base. Mixed-methods approaches allow us to learn about context, process, impact, and outcome, providing evidence on what works, why it works, and in which settings it works best. The need to be able to replicate and increase the scale of an intervention, coupled with advocacy and input into the policy process, are all now important outcomes from an evaluation.

Thus, this third edition starts from a different place. The emphasis has shifted (see Box 1.1). We hope that the book will provide a further contribution to the evidence base, giving a broad perspective to the different types of evidence that are needed, the different methods and approaches to collecting and documenting that evidence, and how to ensure that the results of evaluation make it into the public domain and policy arena.

Box 1.1 The areas of emphasis for evaluating health promotion

- Understanding the processes of implementation and intervention
- Specifics of measurement: tailoring appropriately to the intended outcome
- Building the evidence base incrementally: establishing internal and external validity
- Planning in advance how to influence policy

The scope of health promotion activities

Health has many definitions, ranging from the absence of disease to the concept of enablement or wellbeing, whereas health promotion, in general, has taken its definition from the broader 'wellbeing' end of the spectrum, with a wide range of activities that fit the description of health promotion. Activities related to health promotion can span from providing vaccination to prevent disease at one end of the health spectrum to promotion of social networks at the other (wellbeing) end. Interventions can be focused on individuals, families, schools, communities, or even whole populations. Many models have been proposed to describe the range of interventions that can improve health but few models to date can adequately capture the full extent of activities. The newer social ecological models have shown promise in this direction.

Social ecological models attempt to combine a number of disciplines uniting different areas of research to address the broad definition of health promotion as outlined in the Ottawa Charter (World Health Organization 1986). Social ecological models address the relationships between socio-economic, cultural, political, environmental, organizational, psychological, and biological determinants of health and illness (Stokols *et al.* 1996). For this approach, it is the interplay between people and their settings that is important, and thus social ecological approaches draw on multiple disciplines ranging from epidemiology, psychology, and sociology to therapeutic medicine. Social ecological approaches have been criticized for being too broad, and a solution put forward is to stratify the environment and look for appropriate interventions at each level. The biggest contribution of social ecological models to the further development of health promotion evaluation is that they promote a holistic view of both health and the determinants of health.

Mixed methods are vital to be able to analyse health and the determinants of health at all the different levels they occur. This book provides examples of interventions and evaluations at different levels; for example, from screening for heart disease among individuals (Chapter 13), through mediating community social norms around intimate partner violence (Chapter 9) to managing the physical environment to improve health (Chapter 10) and influencing national policy (Chapter 15).

A different but related approach to social ecology is to consider the range of causal vectors that health promoters might choose to influence in order to increase health and wellbeing. It is well understood in health promotion and in public health that health is determined not just at the individual level but also at a population level, where patterns of health and disease are clearly discernable. Kelly and colleagues (2008) have described four vectors of causation of health at the population level: the *population vector*, in which they include state laws and regulations and the functioning of the economy, the *environmental vector*, including both the natural and built environment, the *organizational vector*, which is 'the framework or the architecture of social life', and the *social vector*, which consists of the cultural and social circumstances of an individual, including deprivation, gender, ethnicity, and so on. As with social ecological approaches, evaluations described in this book include interventions that act on each one of these vectors.

As previously mentioned, few models of health promotion are adequately able to capture the diversity of the discipline and the levels at which it operates. This book provides a range of examples at different levels, in different contexts. It is not within the scope of this book to provide all the possible methods, approaches, and levels at which evaluation can take place. However, our aim has been to highlight the issues and provide examples which may be transferable to other topics and contexts.

Measurement issues in health promotion

The range of activities involved in health promotion, and the multiple levels of operation, generate difficulties for its evaluation and measurement. Each type of activity demands a different form of evaluation. The issue in health promotion evaluation is the accuracy and appropriateness of measurement. This applies equally to quantitative and qualitative study designs. There cannot be just one method for the evaluation of health promotion initiatives because the initiatives themselves draw on a variety of methods and disciplines. The new disciplinary field of mixed methods is very relevant here.

Within this book the issue of measurement is explored primarily in Part II on methods of evaluation. Chapters 4 and 6 focus on experimental designs and systematic reviews and the importance of their contribution to the health promotion evidence base as well as exploring potential problems or areas in which other forms of evidence are needed. This theme is also explored in Chapter 3, which assesses the appropriateness of measurement in terms of outcome and impact. Chapter 3 also considers the level at which outcome measurement should take place and the methods that can be used to build evidence incrementally. Chapter 5 examines the importance of economic evaluation, describing a powerful tool for distinguishing the true value of health promotion interventions as compared to disease treatment.

It is becoming increasingly important to not only measure primary outcomes but to understand how the intervention has brought about this change. Process evaluations, which are described in Chapter 7, are increasingly embedded in study designs and aim both to answer questions about the implementation of the intervention and to place results into context. The importance of context arises throughout the book and is closely related to the understanding and role of validity in evaluation studies.

Internal and external validity

One of the recurring themes of the chapters in this book is the tension between achieving internal validity (through rigorous research designs) to prove the efficacy of an intervention and exploring external validity to understand how effective that intervention might be at a larger scale or in different settings. Understanding the important factors influencing the external validity of an intervention in different settings with different communities is one of the key challenges facing health promotion because of its broad scope, and the many levels at which interventions can take place. Experimental designs and randomized controlled trials (RCTs) in particular, emphasize a strong internal validity. However there is an increasing need to explore, understand, and measure external validity, and this issue is considered in the third section of the book, which explores evaluation in practice.

Chapter 10 on environmental interventions explores how associations between the built environment and health behaviours have been examined and looks at the challenges of and opportunities for evaluating them. Interventions which are context- and setting-specific provide particular challenges to the measurement of both internal and external validity. In Chapter 11, which looks at the use of new information and communications technologies to improve health and health care (e-health), the author discusses the specific issues in the evaluation of online health promotion and the potential benefits of being able to carry out a trial in natural settings thus improving the external validity of interventions.

The importance of context is particularly important in intimate partner violence, the topic of Chapter 9. This chapter, which focuses on the evaluation of interventions to reduce men's use of violence, also shows how mixed-method approaches are necessary to understand the full impact of the intervention on gender-based violence.

A discussion of social marketing (Chapter 8) explores how to improve both internal and external validity of social marketing evaluation through RCT methodology and a thorough exploration of the settings and influences on health at all levels. The chapter also usefully describes the criteria for evaluating and categorizing social marketing interventions.

Ethics and advocacy

The fourth section of this book focuses on the users of and participants in an evaluation. Two recurring themes run through this section: ethics and advocacy. Ethics is explored through interventions designed to empower and involve users in decision-making and action. Advocacy is explored through methods which involve stakeholders in evaluation, dissemination, and the translation of evidence into policy.

Chapter 12 reviews how encouraging and supporting the involvement of lay people in government public health guidance has led to being more responsive and accountable as a public health service. Effective public involvement can contribute to more appropriate policies and services, where decision-making is informed by the experiences of the client group or community and what matters to them.

The complexity of what is meant by 'informed' participation in health promotion activities is discussed in Chapter 13, highlighting some of the ethical considerations needed in health promotion evaluation, and describing how both the content and delivery of information may affect both agreement to participate and participants' satisfaction.

In Chapter 14 the importance of disseminating research findings back to all participants and stakeholders in an evaluation, from both an ethical viewpoint and in order to promote more effective implementation, is reviewed. The feedback of information is an important advocacy tool. Chapter 15 takes this theme one step forward as it investigates ways in which health promotion evaluation can be developed, disseminated, and applied to exert greater policy influence. The emphasis on policy in the last chapter of the book echoes the topic of Chapter 2, where historical and policy approaches to the evaluation of public health and health promotion are described and the importance of understanding the historical precedents of twenty-first-century policy-making is underlined.

This book argues for a broad-minded approach to developing a toolbox of mixed methods for evaluating health promotion in terms of outcomes, impact, and process. Health and wellbeing is present (or may be absent) in many different settings, contexts, and levels. Health can be impacted upon at the individual, community, or societal level. Thus it is also important to include tools that can evaluate interventions at multiple levels and in multiple settings. There is a need to assess both internal and external validity of interventions. The discipline of health promotion must practise good governance ensuring high ethical standards, the development of a robust evidence base, and the provision of evidence that can and will be speedily translated into policy.

Key points

- Mixed-methods approaches which integrate qualitative and quantitative methods are essential to health promotion evaluation.

- The scope of health promotion is vast. No one set of methods or approaches is adequate to deal with the full range of health promotion intervention and determinants of health and wellbeing.

- Measuring interventions appropriately with mixed methods is the key to building a robust evidence base for health promotion.

- Establishing internal and then external validity of interventions helps to build the evidence base incrementally.

- Ensuring good governance and ethics, including multiple stakeholder participation, in evaluation is crucial.

- Evaluation results (whether positive or negative) must be translated into policy in a timely fashion.

References

Craig, P., Dieppe, P., Macintyre, S., Mitchie, S., Nazareth, I., and Petticrew, M. (2008) Developing and evaluating complex interventions: the new Medical Research Council guidance. *British Medical Journal* **337**, 979–83.

Kelly, M., Stewart, E., Morgan, A. *et al.* (2008) A conceptual framework for public health: NICE's emerging approach. *Public Health* **123**(1), e14–20.

Lewin, S., Glenton, C., and Oxman, A.D. (2009) Use of qualitative methods alongside randomised controlled trials of complex healthcare interventions: methodological study. *British Medical Journal* **339**, b3496.

O'Cathain, A., Murphy, E., and Nicholl, J. (2008) The quality of mixed methods studies in health services research. *Journal of Health Services Research and Policy* **13**, 92–8.

Pope, C. and Mays, N. (2009) Critical reflections on the rise of qualitative research. *British Medical Journal* **339**, b3425.

Stokols, D., Allen, J., and Bellingham, R.L. (1996) The social ecology of health promotion – implications for research and practice. *American Journal of Health Promotion* **10**, 247–51.

World Health Organization (1986) *Ottawa Charter for Health Promotion*. World Health Organization & Health and Welfare, Ontario.

Chapter 2

Historical and policy approaches

Virginia Berridge

Public health is an amorphous concept and its meaning to the public is often linked to concerns about sanitation or the environment. The public health 'field' has been bedeviled by arcane discussions about what different terminology for public health really means. One definition has followed another in recent British history; public health, community medicine, prevention, new public health, health promotion. In 2000, the then British health minister, Alan Milburn, showed his irritation with this complexity:

> 'Public health' understood as the epidemiological analysis of the patterns and causes of population health and ill health gets confused with 'public health' understood as population-level health promotion, which in turn gets confused with 'public health' understood as public health professionals trained in medicine.
>
> (Milburn 2000, quoted in Webster and French 2002)

Health promotion, as other chapters in this volume demonstrate, is essentially a fuzzy concept but, for the purposes of this chapter, it is taken to mean the developments since the 1970s whereby the issue of individual health in relation to the environment and social structure has made its way in various forms onto the policy agenda. This chapter will develop a historical understanding of health promotion at two different levels. First, it will look at how what we now term 'health promotion' fits into changing definitions of public health and the rationales for those definitions since the eighteenth century. Then it will carry out an historical evaluation of recent events, looking at how health promotion has come onto the agenda both nationally and internationally since the 1970s.

The long view: changing definitions of public health since the eighteenth century

Nineteenth-century environmentalism

Public health is keen on its historical legacy. The most usual reference point is the nineteenth-century history of public health, the 'heroic' or 'golden' age which provides, so it is argued, an example of environmentalism in action which can speak to present-day international concerns. The spur to reform was epidemic disease, and especially the impact of cholera outbreaks in 1831–2, 1848, and again in the 1860s. The 'hero' of the period (if we are writing heroic history) was Edwin Chadwick, and his famous *Report on the Sanitary Condition of the Labouring Population* (1842). Chadwick drew the link between dirt and disease, and its association with overcrowding and poor sanitation. He called for better water supplies, drainage, and sewage removal. As a follower of Jeremy Bentham's Utilitarian creed, he saw a strong role for the central state to achieve the greatest good for the greatest number. However, Chadwick's practical impact was slight. The Public Health Act of 1848 set up a Central Board of Health. But legislation was only permissive and not compulsory, and there was strong opposition to dictatorship from the centre. Chadwick was removed from his post in 1854 and the Board was abolished. In other industrializing states, however, such conflicts were avoided simply by avoiding the expansion of the central state (Porter 1994).

In Britain, it was at the local level where most was achieved. Sir John Simon, as Medical Officer to the Privy Council Office, helped to push through Public Health Acts in 1872 and 1875 which forced every local authority to establish a sanitary body as well as to inspect housing and monitor food supplies and 'nuisances'. His resignation in 1876 diminished central influence, but local activity still proceeded apace. The Medical Officer of Health, compulsory for the first time at the local level under the 1875 Act, could be a crucial engine of change (Eyler 1997).

There are a number of issues to bear in mind about the nineteenth-century story. First is the nature of the links between poverty and ill health. Chadwick was Secretary to the Poor Law Commission and his concern for health reform arose out of the concern for pauperism. Ill health caused poverty and therefore a possible reliance on the parish and poor relief. This was the human capital approach to health reform, a response which has often been replicated since. The term social capital in contemporary health promotion recalls this legacy. Public health reform was a surrogate and replacement in nineteenth-century England for more general social reform (Hamlin 1998).

This is a British story and the details of these developments were not universally replicated in all countries. Dorothy Porter has pointed out, for example, that industrialization was not a necessary prerequisite for central government intervention in health; nor was the centralization model automatically adopted by states. Forms of public health were clearly dependent on the history and cultures of particular countries (Porter 1994). In other European countries, public health was a more radical creed. Rudolf Virchow and other public health doctors were supporters of the 1848 revolutions across Europe and their programme was one of social and political action.

The question also arises of how much impact public health interventions really had. This has been a long-running debate among historical demographers which has implications for those who plan and run health services in the contemporary world. The so-called McKeown thesis, that formal medical interventions actually achieved little and that rising living standards achieved more, has been challenged by a view which gives a greater role for formal public health in the nineteenth century (Szreter 1988).

It is important to remember, too, how the impetus behind public health was informed by fear. Fear was focused on what was seen as the growth of a 'residuum', a race of degenerates, physically stunted and morally inferior. The residuum was seen as an agent of infection, both of healthy bodies and of the body politic. Dirt was considered to be dangerous not only at the individual level, but also at the political level. This larger ideological climate for reform was connected with the concern for environmental pollution of the late nineteenth century, when the fear of contamination crossed boundaries of social and health concern. It is from this period that we derive our images of the fog-shrouded East End of London.

Bacteriology and personal prevention

In the twentieth century, the ideology of public health changed and its focus narrowed. Winslow, an American public health authority, identified three phases in the development of public health: the first, from 1840 to 1890, was characterized by environmental sanitation; the second, from 1890 to 1910, by developments in bacteriology, resulting in an emphasis on isolation and disinfection; and the third, beginning around 1910, by an emphasis on education and personal hygiene, referred to as personal prevention.

Let us take bacteriology first. The discoveries of Koch and Pasteur in the late nineteenth century made public health more important as a profession: it was now possible to pinpoint specific causes of disease and bacteriology soon came to dominate the public health curriculum. But at another level, these developments moved the focus of attention away from the environment and towards the individual patient as the locus of infection. In fact, some historians have argued that these theories gained widespread acceptability quickly at the political level precisely because they provided such a circumscribed notion of appropriate intervention. Others have drawn attention to how the terminology of germs was used and only gave way to bacteria after the 1880s. Public health practice could be at odds with theory, although a linear model of innovation was presented publicly (Worboys 2000). At the same time, governments took up the issue of social welfare reform through universal education, pensions, health insurance, and school meals, and so the barriers between health and social reform became higher and more impermeable.

Some historians and sociologists argue that bacteriology had a negligible effect on the implementation of policy. Its importance lay in preparing the way for the rise of what has been called 'surveillance medicine' (Armstrong 1983). The new public health of the early twentieth century was indeed founded on the concept of 'personal prevention'. This was also a marriage between public health and eugenics. The political imperative for reform was there, especially after the Boer War had revealed the shortcomings of British army recruits and heightened eugenic fears of 'national deterioration' and 'racial decline'. But the focus was on the individual, and especially the individual mother.

The concept of 'maternal efficiency' was prevalent. Lewis (1980) has pointed to the tensions implicit in the way the infant mortality rate was conceived of as a problem of maternal ignorance. The death rate was highest in poor inner-city slums, where unsanitary living conditions prevailed. Yet public health doctors and civil servants tended to see maternal and child health as a question of providing health visitors, personal services, and health education. Mothers were encouraged to breast-feed and to achieve higher standards of domestic hygiene. The possibility of rising living standards and real wages during the First World War may have had more impact on the infant mortality rate, but public health came increasingly to mean the delivery of personal health services.

The interwar years in the UK: new tendencies

In the 1920s and 1930s, the interwar years, public health went down divergent routes and the gulf between practice and theory widened. The case study of the UK illustrates some of the dangers which public health as an occupation can be prey to. This was a golden age in one sense for public health as an occupation. Public health doctors were running a wide range of services at the local level. When local government took on the administration of Poor Law hospitals after 1929, many public health doctors found themselves running those hospitals. The range of services under the public health umbrella in these interwar years was huge, especially in London, where the municipal hospital system was one of the most extensive in the world. But there was conflict for territory at the local level with the general practitioner, the primary family physician. How did public health doctors differ from general practitioners? The local authority clinic, home of the Medical Officer of Health, seemed to many general practitioners to be offering only what they could also provide through their individual practices. Some historians have concluded that this administrative expansion was achieved only at the expense of the neglect of the 'community watchdog' role of the Medical Officer of Health (Webster 1982) but more recent research has concluded that public health performed well at the local level, although the picture was variable, with different responses in different localities (Levene *et al.* 2004).

The cutting intellectual edge of public health lay outside the discipline, in particular through the work of academics in social medicine, who remained distinct from public health practitioners. Social medicine ideas that took a more holistic view of health were advocated by Richard Titmuss, John Ryle, and others in the UK. This was also an international movement which had its advocates and initiatives in many countries throughout the world. The work of Henry Sigerist in the USA and Rene Sand in Belgium was paralleled by that of the social medicine movement in South Africa, exemplified in the work of the Karks in primary health care (Porter 1999, Solomon *et al.* 2008). The Peckham Health Centre in the 1930s in south London also exemplified a new view of health which encompassed social wellbeing as well as intervention to treat disease.

The recent view: new definitions and the rise of health promotion

In the post-war years, public health underwent redefinition and realignment structurally. In the UK public health doctors lost their administrative 'empires'. At the same time a reorientation of public health focus towards the modification of individual lifestyle took place. Then changes on the international scene brought the arrival of the new approach, termed health promotion.

Post-war failure and realignment

The traditional service-based view of public health ran into the sand in post-war Britain. Public health, contrary to the expectations of many in the profession, did not form the basis of a reformed health service. Public health doctors lost their hospital role, and faced a decline in clinic work because of the universal access provided to the general practitioner. The NHS was set up as a 'sickness service' rather than one which emphasized positive health. The local authority role was also under strain with the desire of parts of the public health empire—sanitary inspectors, social workers—to break away. The notion of 'community medicine', of the public health doctor as health strategist, arose at this time. Jerry Morris at the London School of Hygiene and Tropical Medicine (LSHTM) first defined such work as based on the principles of epidemiology: the community physician would be responsible for 'community diagnosis' and therefore the effective administration of health services. This was the vision put into practice through the policy documents of the late 1960s: the Seebohm Committee and the Todd Commission on Medical Education. Community physicians were to be the linchpin of the NHS, linking all aspects of lay and medical administration (Lewis 1986). They were to be both advisers and managers. In practice, these roles were difficult to juggle. There were tensions between the responsibility to the community outside the hospital and the accountability to the health authority. After health service reorganization in the 1980s community medicine virtually disappeared.

Lifestyle and individual behaviour as public health

Parallel to this administrative change in the UK, a more general reorientation of public health towards concepts of lifestyle and behaviour began to take place. The roots of this reorientation can be traced to the research in the 1940s and 1950s which linked smoking with the rise in lung cancer. These scientific discoveries represented a fundamental paradigm shift in scientific ways of knowing. For biomedical theories of direct causation they substituted the epidemiological notion of relative risk and statistical correlation (Berridge 2007). Epidemiology became the new public health/preventive medicine discipline par excellence, associated with a whole host of health issues, from alcohol and smoking through to diet, exercise, and heart disease. This was the epitome of the surveillance society. A public health agenda emerged in the 1960s and 1970s which was based on individual avoidance of risk. It developed a strong economic dimension (the human capital arguments of the nineteenth century revisited), and a focus on education of the individual. Consequently the role of health education assumed new significance. Techniques of mass persuasion began to be widely used in the health arena from the 1960s and 1970s.

Criticism of this approach came from a variety of directions. Some saw the emphasis on individual responsibility for health as a political ploy to divert attention from the real socio-economic causes of disease and the failures of health care systems. These condemned the 'victim-blaming' and 'sickness as sin' arguments implicit within preventive health.

The individual-responsibility argument divorced the person from the social environment. Criticism came also from an entirely different direction; from the 'Radical Right' which argued that government wished to institute what it called the 'nanny state' where habits which should be left to individual discretion were regulated and controlled unnecessarily (Le Fanu 1994). Proponents of this line of argument often called attention to the fragility of the scientific arguments supporting particular preventive policies. Prevention was crucially about the reduction of statistical risk to the community as a whole, not, as in curative medicine, about delivering benefits to identifiable individuals. In surveys where the public ranked different medical and health interventions, medical technology ranked high whereas lifestyle efforts received lower levels of public support.

The rise of smoking as an issue most clearly epitomised the reorientation of public health towards individual lifestyle. By the 1970s, anti-smoking interests had developed a policy agenda which focused on economic argument (price and tax rises, anti-industry) and on the media (advertising bans, mass-media campaigns), sustained through the techniques of epidemiology (Berridge 2007). In the 1980s, the development of HIV/AIDS as an issue also epitomised many of those public health concerns. AIDS was a syndrome initially defined solely via epidemiology and through the concept of risk. AIDS was an epidemiological syndrome par excellence; and it also seemed to exemplify the key tenets of the new public health, stressing modification of individual behaviour and individual responsibility rather than any collective reaction (Berridge 1996, Leichter 1991). In the policy responses favoured by western liberal democracies—behaviour modification and health education campaigns—it exemplified the lifestyle approach.

Health promotion as an international movement

Alongside lifestyle, a broader approach to health began to emerge, termed health promotion. This had contextual roots in common with lifestyle public health. As Webster and French (2002) have pointed out, social medicine had become an international movement, with influence in the USA and at the World Health Organization (WHO). The radical critique of medicine gathered pace through the very different approaches of Thomas McKeown, Archie Cochrane's *Effectiveness and Efficiency*, and the writings of Ivan Ilich and Thomas Szasz. The shortcomings of models of health focused only on the provision of health services—in particular hospital-based services—became apparent, especially in developing countries. Allied with this was a realization of the rising costs of such models of health care and the impact of the oil price rise imposed by Organization of Petroleum-Exporting Countries (OPEC) states at the end of 1973 (Webster and French 2002).

Health promotion as it emerged had what David McQueen has called a 'Canadian European' focus (McQueen 2008). Canada was a central initial location with the publication of the Lalonde Report in 1974 (MacDougall 2007). The impetus came also through the international primary health care movement, the Declaration of Alma Ata (1978) and the goal of Health for All in the year 2000. The Declaration of Alma Ata advocated an intersectoral and multidimensional approach to health and socio-economic development, emphasized the use of appropriate technology, and urged active community participation in health care and health education at every level (Cueto 2004). In 1986, at a conference held in Ottawa, under the leadership of the WHO and with strong support from its Director General, Halfdan Mahler, the Charter for Health Promotion was adopted. The Ottawa Charter moved the focus of public health from disease prevention to 'capacity building for health'. It was tied through the work of the Pan American Health Organization (PAHO) and the European office of the WHO (WHO-Euro) to an approach which moved beyond health care to a commitment to social reform and equity (Kickbusch 2003).

The work of WHO-Euro was important in carrying forward this broader vision. In WHO-Euro 38 Health for All targets were adopted in 1984. The WHO Regional Committee had taken the stance that lifestyles need to be understood as collective behaviours rooted in context. Ann Taket, who was a consultant in the WHO regional office in 1983–4, has conveyed the sense of excitement and the tensions apparent during this period (Berridge *et al.* 2006). Social scientists like the sociologist Margaret Stacey and the health economist Brian Abel Smith were advisers and the work had the support of the regional director Jo Asvall. The Health Education Unit at WHO-Euro was led by a sociologist, Ilona Kickbusch, and its programme dealt with lay, community, and alternative health care; public education and information for health; health promotion; and smoking. This thinking was very different to a second major influence on the work of the regional office, the management by objective approach which focused on individual behaviour modification. There was a sense of 'watching two worlds collide' with tensions between the technician and activist outlooks and between medical and non-medical world views (Berridge *et al.* 2006).

The history of health promotion in the USA was different. In that country, health promotion remained more closely tied to health education and structurally to chronic disease prevention. The USA remained wedded to a narrower view. WHO-Euro developed the 'settings' approach which focused on creating networks. The Regional Office began to work with local authorities, cities, universities, organizations, hospitals, and schools to carry forward the new message in what Kickbusch has called an 'international learning process'. In 1987, the Healthy Cities project was launched explicitly to bypass national health ministries and aimed at localizing health promotion, building a strong lobby at the local level (Petersen and Lupton 1996). In Liverpool in England a regional health promotion group developed in the Mersey Regional Health Authority and Howard Seymour was recruited as the country's first Regional Health Promotion Officer. Coinciding with concern about expanding drug use and the arrival of HIV/AIDS, this gave health promotion impetus at the local level. The health promoter Jeff French's recollection was that the 1980s and 1990s were an exciting time when health promotion practitioners were increasing in number and were action-oriented. But 'old public health' attempted to subvert the new discipline of health promotion, first by redefining it as a subset of mainstream public health and then by the promotion of a new set of activities called the 'new public health' (Berridge *et al.* 2006). Some argued that 'new public health' was simply a medical tactic to regain control of the public health agenda from health promotion interests, who were far from exclusively medical. The subsequent rise of multidisciplinary public health in the UK saw the integration of health promotion practitioners within the public health profession in the UK and the change from public health as a medical-only occupation (Evans and Knight 2006).

Historical evaluation

Historical evaluation of public health and health promotion does not set out to give some of the answers traditionally associated with the process of evaluation. It cannot tell us what works best, what is cost-effective, or which intervention to put in place, or advise us on the best technique for assessment. Rather this chapter has tried to point out how health promotion is a component of a public health history which traces its origins to the desire of states to deal with issues of human capital. Behavioural rather than structural explanations have dominated in twentieth century history. But health promotion in its European version has tried to focus on what Ryle in 1948 called the 'whole economic, nutritional, occupational, educational and psychological opportunity or experience of the individual or community'. Tensions with different conceptions of public health have continued and health promotion has also been at the mercy, in the British context, of continuing structural reorganization. The contested nature of public health and its definitions reflects the tensions within the world in which it has to operate.

Key points

- Public health is not an unchanging concept but has gone through different formulations since the nineteenth century.
- The nineteenth-century definitions of public health focused initially on environmentalism and sanitarianism; and then on bacteriology and personal prevention.
- Public health can be seduced by administrative responsibilities. In the UK it was at the height of its administrative power in the interwar years, but historians are debating how effective it really was. Current research presents a more positive picture.

- Social medicine, as the academic version of public health, began to develop a more holistic attitude to health.
- Lifestyle and risk factors dominated in post-war public health, epitomized by smoking.
- Health promotion arose out of Canadian and European influence and also the primary health care movement, which had a particular focus on the developing world.
- Health promotion's influence was strongly local and community-based, but was challenged by a 'new public health' which was more medicalized. Such tensions and the 'fuzziness' of health promotion still remain.

References

Armstrong, D. (1983) *Political Anatomy of the Body. Medical Knowledge in Britain in the Twentieth Century.* Cambridge University Press, Cambridge.

Berridge, V. (1996) *AIDS in the UK: the Making of Policy, 1981–1994.* Oxford University Press, Oxford.

Berridge, V. (2007) *Marketing Health. Smoking and the Discourse of Public Health in Britain, 1945–2000.* Oxford University Press, Oxford.

Berridge, V., Christie, D., and Tansey, E.M. (2006) *Public Health in the 1980s and 1990s: Decline and Rise? Wellcome Witnesses to Twentieth Century Medicine,* volume **26**. Wellcome Trust Centre for the History of Medicine, London. www.ucl.ac.uk/histmed/publications/wellcome_witnesses_c20th_med/vol_26.

Cueto, M. (2004) The origins of primary health care and selective primary health care. *American Journal of Public Health* **94**(11), 1864–74.

Evans, D. and Knight, T. (2006) *There was no Plan! –The Origins and Development of Multi Disciplinary Public Health in the UK.* Faculty of Health and Social Care, University of the West of England, Bristol. http://hsc.uwe.ac.uk/net/research/Data/Sites/1/GalleryImages/Research/History_of_MDPH_Witness_Seminar_Report.pdf.

Eyler, J. (1997) *Sir Arthur Newsholme and State Medicine, 1885–1935.* Cambridge University Press, Cambridge.

Hamlin, C. (1998) *Public Health and Social Justice in the Age of Chadwick. Britain, 1800–1854.* Cambridge University Press, Cambridge.

Kickbusch, I. (2003) The contribution of the World Health Organization to a new public health and health promotion. *American Journal of Public Health* **93**(3), 383–8.

Le Fanu, J. (1994) *Preventionitis. The exaggerated Claims of Health Promotion.* Social Affairs Unit, London.

Leichter, H. (1991) *Free to be Foolish. Politics and Health Promotion in the United States and Great Britain.* Princeton University Press, Princeton, NJ.

Levene, A., Powell, M., and Stewart, J. (2004) Patterns of municipal health expenditure in inter war England and Wales. *Bulletin of the History of Medicine* **78** (3), 635–69.

Lewis, J. (1980) *The Politics of Motherhood. Child and Maternal Welfare in England, 1900–1939.* Croom Helm, London.

Lewis, J. (1986) *What Price Community Medicine?* Harvester, Brighton.

MacDougall, H. (2007) Reinventing public health: a new perspective on the health of Canadians and its international impact. *Journal of Epidemiology and Community Health* **61**, 955–9.

McQueen, D.V. (2008) Self reflections on health promotion in the UK and the USA. *Public Health* **122**, 1035–7.

Petersen, A. and Lupton, D. (1996) *The New Public Health. Health and Self in an Age of Risk.* Sage, London.

Porter, D. (1994) *The History of Public Health and the Modern State.* Rodopi, Amsterdam.

Porter, D. (1999) *Health, Civilisation and the State: a History of Public Health from Ancient to Modern Times.* Routledge, London.

Solomon, S.G., Murard, L., and Zylberman, P. (2008) *Shifting Boundaries of Pubic Health. Europe in the Twentieth Century.* University of Rochester Press, Rochester, NY.

Szreter, S. (1988) The importance of social intervention in Britain's mortality decline, c.1850–1914: a reinterpretation of the role of public health. *Social History of Medicine* **1**(1), 1–37.

Webster, C. (1982) Healthy or hungry thirties? *History Workshop Journal* **13**, 110–29.

Webster, C. and French, J. (2002) The cycle of conflict: the history of the public health and health promotion movements. In L. Adams, M. Amos, and J. Munro, eds, *Promoting Health. Politics and Practice*, pp. 5–12. Sage, London.

Worboys, M. (2000) *Spreading Germs. Disease Theories and Medical Practice in Britain, 1865–1900.* Cambridge University Press, Cambridge.

Part II

Methods of evaluation

Chapter 3

Evaluating according to purpose and resources: strengthening the evidence base incrementally

Yolande Coombes

It is acknowledged that for health promotion to remain credible as a discipline it must be evidence-based and to achieve this there has to be rigorous evaluation (Nutbeam 1999, Raphael 2000). However, all too often a potentially useful project is abandoned because the 'gold standards' of experimental designs cannot be attained to evaluate it; in the process a lot of useful information is lost or overlooked that might have also contributed to strengthening the evidence base for health promotion. Our desire for quick fixes and rapid improvement mean that there is tendency to want evaluations that answer definitive questions with certainty. However, evidence in any field rarely comes from just one source, and often the smallest pieces of evidence incrementally add up to the strongest case. We must be careful in our search for evidence and the need to evaluate that we do not confuse small-scale or incremental evaluation with poor evaluation.

Strengthening the evidence base for health promotion

We need the results of evaluations to inform evidence-based decision-making. Evaluation allows us to:

- compare efficiency and cost-effectiveness, which are central to the development of new initiatives;

- assess and assure the quality of an intervention or project over time;
- ensure that interventions are effective as well as efficacious, in that they can be replicated in different settings and under different conditions (see Chapter 4 in this volume for a discussion of effectiveness and efficacy);
- replicate and scale up an intervention.

The main problem faced, is in deciding what counts as evidence. Part of the problem arises from the differences in how health is defined and how its impact is measured. Health in the context of health promotion is usually defined as 'a resource for everyday living' or 'complete mental, physical, spiritual and emotional wellbeing, not just the absence of disease', yet evidence is usually taken in the form of a reduction in mortality or morbidity (Raphael 2000). The social, economic, and emotional determinants of health are often overlooked in the search for evidence for effectiveness which fit a more biomedical approach to health and health promotion (see Chapter 2 on views of health and public health). McQueen (2001) suggests that evidence in health promotion does not really come from health promotion as a complete discipline itself but from the effectiveness of specific disciplinary subcomponents of the health promotion intervention. This leads to health promotion being reduced to its component parts and rarely being evaluated in a holistic sense, which is how the discipline defines itself. For example, health promotion interventions tend to concentrate on physical health gain (one subcomponent) much more than social, economic, or emotional health gain. It is unusual to find an evaluation which evaluates health in its entirety.

Enough evidence exists to justify health promotion as a discipline that can improve the health of the population. In a recent editorial Catford (2009) argued that 'the tide has turned with mounting evidence of the value and cost–benefit of health promotion'; he cites evidence from treasury reports in the UK, Australia, and the USA. But Catford also calls for more evidence on the effectiveness of how health promotion is delivered. It is not enough to know whether an intervention is cost-effective in a trial situation; we need evidence about how easy or hard it is to carry out that same intervention at large scale, and not in an experimental context. Similarly, Raphael (2000) argues that although there is ample evidence concerning the impact of interventions on the determinants of health in experimental situations, what is needed is more accumulated evidence to see whether interventions have been effective in real settings where there is no experimental influence (see Chapter 10, which examines interventions in natural settings).

There will always be a role for large-scale evaluation studies on intervention efficacy but evidence takes many forms and the applicability and effectiveness of interventions in the context of everyday lives—the context within which health takes place—should be given more prominence. More than a decade ago, Tones (1997) argued that instead of trying to achieve evidence from one source we should follow the format of a judicial review where we can accept evidence even where 100% proof is not available. Combining this point with the need for evaluation in the local context suggests a need for different types of evaluations at all levels, focused on particular contexts to build a more holistic picture of health promotion.

McQueen (2001), in citing a guide to evidence for health promotion (see Box 3.1), suggests that evaluation need not cover all these

Box 3.1 Definition of evidence for health promotion

The definition of the term 'evidence for health promotion' given by the US Center for Disease Control includes (Briss *et al.* 2000, p.36):

+ information that is appropriate for answering questions about an intervention's effectiveness;

+ the applicability of effectiveness data (i.e. the extent to which available effectiveness data are thought to apply to additional populations and settings);

+ the intervention's positive or negative side effects;

+ economic impact;

+ barriers to implementation of interventions.

five points, but that each or all of them contribute to the evidence base. Thus a small-scale evaluation concentrating on the process of implementation makes an equally important contribution to our evidence as a large-scale trial looking at efficacy. Nutbeam (1999) argues that given the complexity of health promotion interventions there can be no 'absolute' form of evidence and no 'right' method of evaluation. He suggests that evidence for effectiveness is linked to the entry point of the evaluation and the intervention. McQueen (2001) echoes this by saying that as the complexity of an intervention increases we need more complicated methods of assessment, and that answers provided by that assessment may be less clear.

Evidence as outcomes

The need for 'evidence' to prove the effectiveness of an intervention is now almost synonymous with the 'outcomes' that are measured, hence the emphasis on outcome evaluation. To measure outcomes from an intervention necessitates a certain degree of precision in measurement, and often considerable resources. A randomized controlled trial (RCT) will provide internally valid evidence of effectiveness. Well-designed RCTs may also have some external validity but the RCT is not without its limitations (see Chapters 4–6, which examine the hierarchy of evidence and the role of RCTs), particularly within health promotion where random allocation of individuals or communities to experimental and control groups is not always possible. But, more importantly, we need to know whether an intervention works in the 'real' world, not just in experimental settings. Green and Tones (1999, p.134) note that:

> . . .health promotion is frequently a multifactoral intervention having a range of possible outcomes. Experimental designs that would fully accommodate this intricacy, with the capacity to discriminate between different components of the intervention, would inevitably be highly complex, involve sophisticated analytic techniques, very large samples – and ipso facto, exceed the budgetary constraints of most programmes.

Some health promotion interventions are attempting to measure different components of an intervention with hard (morbidity and mortality) outcomes in real-world settings (see case study 2 in Box 3.3).

But these types of intervention are rare, because of the associated high costs of evaluation. So how can we solve the issue of needing evidence within the 'real' context?

To answer this question we need to go back to the issue of whether biomedical health outcomes are, or should be, the only type of evidence that we accept. Green and Jones (1999) point out the inadequacy of relying solely on changes in morbidity and mortality as outcome measures of an intervention. Instead they turn the argument on its head. They suggest that health promotion interventions should only be developed if they can be based on existing demonstrated evidence that the intervention will have impact on morbidity and mortality. Therefore, hard outcomes provide the justification for developing interventions and not the means of evaluating their effect.

We need large-scale evaluation with hard outcome measures of morbidity and mortality to provide firm evidence, but these studies tend to be experimental in design and so are rarely applicable in real-world settings. Because we need to evaluate how interventions are implemented in the real world, we need evaluations which are more focused on process and method (the inputs) and not just the outcomes.

Evaluating outcome measures over time

Outcome measures change over time. Nutbeam (1998) discusses the concept of outcome hierarchies which emphasize the difference between short-term impact and longer-term health outcomes. At one end of this continuum immediate changes of effectiveness are characterized by changes in knowledge or skills of individuals. This moves through changes in the determinants of health, health behaviours, and socio-economic and environmental conditions through to, at the far end of the continuum, changes in health outcomes in terms of morbidity and mortality.

Green and Tones (1999) also use this concept of indicators of success along a continuum and point to changes in proximal indicators as being more likely to be due to the impact of the intervention than changes in distal indicators, which may take many years to develop. They give the example of 40 years or so for a school-based

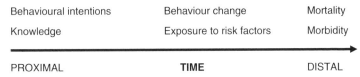

Fig. 3.1 Outcome measures changing over time

smoking-cessation programme to have an effect on the incidence of lung cancer. They therefore reject epidemiological indicators for evaluating health promotion and instead say that the focus of attention should be on the psychosocial and environmental factors that influence health and health-related decision-making, for which we have an increased theoretical understanding from a number of explanatory models. They suggest that the use of these models allows the various stages along the continuum from proximal to distal to be defined, and those most proximal to be selected for evaluation (see Chapter 8, which outlines how this can be done for the evaluation of social marketing interventions). Figure 3.1 outlines how we might examine different outcome measures over time.

The advantage of this continuum perspective is that where links between indicators at different points on the continuum have already been evaluated and established there is no need demonstrate the relationship again, and therefore our evaluation efforts should be concentrated on the relationships between indicators where the evidence is less well established (Green and Tones 1999).

What this type of evaluation shows us (in Box 3.2) is that evidence can be built incrementally. Our goal is to reduce the incidence and prevalence of HIV/AIDS. We know this can be done through reducing the number of sexual partners, abstinence, mutual faithfulness, and consistent condom use. We already have the evidence on some of the determinants of safer sex behaviour. Therefore to evaluate the intervention we do not need to evaluate at the level of reductions in morbidity or mortality, or even at the level of reductions in incidence or prevalence. The evaluation can be at the level of demonstrating changes in personal risk perception (as measured by trust, caution and received assurances) and associated changes in exposure to risk factors and behaviour change.

Box 3.2 Case study 1. Trust and caution; ways to reduce HIV

Population Services International (PSI), through AIDSMARK funding, ran a campaign across several countries in East and Southern Africa to increase personal risk perception of HIV/AIDS with the aim of increasing safer sex behaviours. This campaign sought to increase caution and received assurances between partners (such as agreeing on mutual faithfulness or voluntary counselling and testing (VCT)), maintaining interpersonal trust while reducing sexual trust. We already know that safer sex behaviour is related to a cluster of psychological, social, and environmental influences, including beliefs about the benefits of safer sex behaviours outweighing barriers; self-efficacy to negotiate condom use or discuss partner assurances; availability of condoms; and personal risk perception. The PSI programme evaluated changes in these indicators in addition to changes in trust, caution, and received assurances (see Figure 3.2). At a more distal level, reported sexual behaviour was evaluated, including reduction in partners, consistent condom use, and uptake of VCT. The furthest distal changes in HIV-positive incidence were not evaluated because they were too difficult to attribute to the campaign and were too difficult to measure given the resources available (Klein and Coombes 2005).

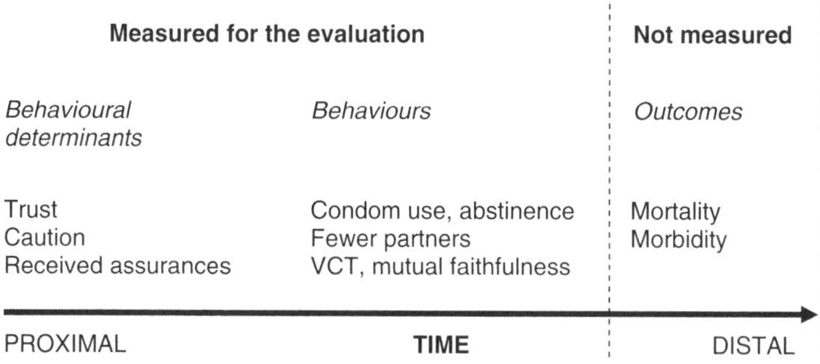

Measured for the evaluation		Not measured
Behavioural determinants	*Behaviours*	*Outcomes*
Trust	Condom use, abstinence	Mortality
Caution	Fewer partners	Morbidity
Received assurances	VCT, mutual faithfulness	
PROXIMAL	**TIME**	DISTAL

Fig. 3.2 Outcome measures for the Population Services International (PSI) personal risk perception/trusted partner campaign
VCT, voluntary counselling and testing.

Using this incremental approach to evaluation we are able to build evidence along the causal chain and from a combination of real-world and experimental settings. Each level of outcome evaluation on the proximal–distal continuum utilizes different indicators of measurement from behavioural determinants at the proximal end through to changes in mortality at the distal end (see Box 3.3 for further examples of this).

Determining the level of outcome measures and the method of evaluation

We have established that incremental gains in evidence from different levels of evaluation contribute to the health promotion evidence base. But how do you decide what level of outcome to measure and what type of evaluation is needed? To define this we first need to answer the question: why are we evaluating? Habicht *et al.* (1999) argue that this question is seldom discussed yet is fundamental to choosing an appropriate evaluation design. They suggest that the main objective of any evaluation is to influence decisions; therefore, how complex and precise the evaluation must be depends on who the decision-maker is and what types of decisions will be taken as a consequence of the findings. Both complex and simple evaluations should be equally rigorous in relating the evaluation design to the decisions. These arguments are similar to Andreasen's (1985) backwards research process, which is based on the premise that a researcher should first decide what decisions are going to be made on the basis of research findings and work backwards from that point to design research.

The decisions that will be taken also determine the level of evaluation. We can distinguish four broad levels of evaluation—process, adequacy, plausibility, and probability—that can provide the required level of evidence along our proximal–distal continuum of evaluation outcome evidence.

- **Process** Process evaluation is an essential component of any impact or outcome evaluation or can be an evaluation in itself. Process evaluation is about measuring the inputs of an intervention: how it was carried out. Therefore process evaluation is an end in itself when the importance of real-world settings and the need for better understanding of implementation is

Box 3.3 Case study 2. Scaling up sanitation

Evidence already exists about the role of improved sanitation in reducing diarrhoeal disease morbidity and mortality (Fewtrell *et al.* 2005). Most of that evidence is from experimental trials. In order to achieve millennium development goals for sanitation the Bill and Melinda Gates Foundation have funded a project through the Water and Sanitation Program of the World Bank (<http://www.wsp.org>) designed to learn about effective implementation at scale. Accordingly the project, which is taking place in India, Indonesia, and Tanzania, has four main objectives.

1. The first is to increase the improved sanitation coverage through developing large-scale and sustained *demand* for improved sanitation.

2. The second is to simultaneously *supply* the demand with appropriate products and services, and create large-scale sustainable and effective supply of sanitation and hygiene services and products.

3. The third is to learn the most effective approaches to scaling up and sustaining sanitation programmes including the optimum ways to do the above, and how to replicate in other contexts.

4. The fourth is strengthening knowledge and understanding of health, economic, and social impacts of large-scale sustainable sanitation programs.

To meet these objectives several different evaluation components have been designed. At the highest level of outcomes, a large-impact evaluation study will be undertaken using a randomized experimental approach. However, the evaluation includes other components such as a management information system (to measure inputs) and measures of the enabling environment (the local political, economic, and social systems and infrastructure) and how it impacts on scaling up improved sanitation at district and national levels.

Box 3.3 Case study 2. Scaling up sanitation *(cont)*

A tracking survey over several time points is planned to provide evidence for programme decision-making during the course of the interventions so that the effectiveness of the activities can be monitored. Monitoring analysis provides evidence of trends over time in exposure to the interventions and progress on key indicators such as behaviour and behavioural determinants.

The combination of an RCT, measurement of inputs from the management information system, the enabling environment measures, and a tracking survey will allow the project team to accurately pinpoint exactly what their outcomes were and how they achieved them, which should allow others to replicate and scale up similar projects. An RCT on its own would not answer the objectives; similarly, none of the individual components of the evaluation would be sufficient on their own. However, when brought together the evaluation of this project should provide a significant step forward for the implementation of sanitation programmes.

---

acknowledged. Process evaluation is one level lower than adequacy assessment, but should also be a component of adequacy, plausibility, and probability assessment criteria (see Chapter 7 for a further discussion of process evaluation).

◆ **Adequacy** Did the expected changes occur? This is the cheapest and easiest form of evaluation; it requires no control group as long as results are compared with pre-set criteria, most usually set out in an intervention-logical framework. However, if adequacy is to be measured over time then at least two measurements will be required, increasing the complexity of the evaluation. It is not possible to link adequacy measures to intervention activities but they can provide reassurance that expected goals are being met. This leads us back to the question of why the evaluation is being carried out or what decision will be made on the basis of the evaluation. If the decision to be taken is about continued support for a programme or intervention then adequacy assessment may be all that is needed.

◆ **Plausibility** Did the intervention seem to have an effect above and beyond other external influences? Plausibility assessment is needed where the decision-makers require a greater degree of confidence that any observed changes were in fact due to the intervention. Plausibility assessment tries to rule out external factors and requires rigorous study designs to control for confounding factors.

◆ **Probability** Finally at the level of probability assessment, the answer is being sought to the question 'Did the intervention have an effect ($P<X\%$)?'. Evaluation at this level needs a far more rigorous research design, utilizing RCTs or longitudinal study designs.

Taking Andreasen's (1985) backwards research process and applying it to evaluation and the level of required decision-making and evaluation we come up with the flowchart shown in Figure 3.3.

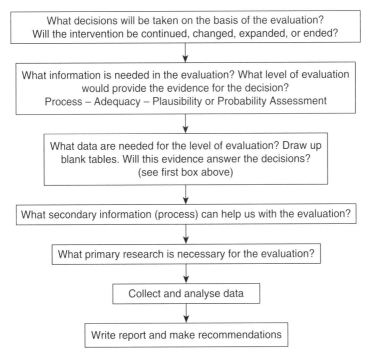

Fig. 3.3 The backwards evaluation process

In summary, evaluation in terms of outcomes can take place on a continuum. Depending on how much evidence we already have on the relationship between different indicators on that continuum determines the level of our outcome evaluation. Secondly, our level of evaluation should be focused on what decisions will be taken on the basis of the evaluation: this helps us to determine the level of adequacy, plausibility, or probability that we need to make, and thus feeds back into the evaluation design. It is essential to design the level of evaluation at the outset of the intervention design, during the initial planning phase, in order to determine the nature and type of evaluation and the associated resources that will be needed. However, it is possible that following this backwards evaluation process, even at the planning stage, might lead to the conclusion that there are not enough resources to carry out the required level of evaluation. What then?

Evaluation in resource-poor settings

Realizing that you do not have sufficient resources for the required level of evaluation is most likely where new causal pathways between an intervention and distal outcome are being hypothesized; in other words, where the evidence base is weak. There are two options. The first is to abandon the intervention until adequate resources for the evaluation can be found. The second is to move the outcome measurement to a more proximal level and use the evaluation as one incremental step in the evidence base.

In addition to revising the evaluation to more proximal indicators, valuable evidence can be gained from process evaluation. Health promotion needs to learn more about the process of implementation—how we deliver health promotion—in natural (rather than experimental) settings to strengthen the external validity of interventions. For interventions to be adopted and disseminated to other locations, it is essential that the process and inputs have been evaluated adequately. The process of implementation can be captured using both quantitative and qualitative data to capture the diversity and detail of implementation, so that the evidence gathered from evaluating the implementation process becomes part of the cycle of evidence into practice (Speller 2005).

Where interventions are being rolled out after their efficacy and effectiveness is established, evaluation should focus on process and implementation issues which can be carried out with minimal resources. Documenting thoroughly how the intervention is designed and implemented and keeping good cost and activity data in a simple management information system can allow a programme to be evaluated against other similar programmes (including those where the evidence for the intervention came from). It all goes back to the question of what decisions will be taken on the basis of the evaluation.

In summary, the evidence base for health promotion is increasing all the time. There is a tendency to try to evaluate outcomes at the highest level in order for them to be considered 'evidence'. However, evidence can also be pieced together incrementally and there is a significant role for evaluations that are focused on the context of implementation. Outcome evaluation occurs on a continuum and interventions can focus their evaluation on those outcomes closest to the intervention, especially where there is already evidence for the existence of a relationship between indicators and outcomes. The key question to be asked is how will the evaluation be used: what is its purpose and what decisions will be made? By following a backwards evaluation process we can conserve our resources and aim for an evaluation that will answer the required questions and contribute to the evidence base. Finally, even when resources do not permit outcome evaluation, process evaluation in its simplest form can help to improve the intervention and can still contribute to the evidence base.

Key points

- There is a huge body of evidence for the effectiveness of health promotion.
- The evidence base can be contributed to in an incremental way from small-scale process evaluations through to hard-outcome RCTs, combining different sorts of evaluation. Thus different types of evidence can make the strongest case.

- Morbidity and mortality data provide the justification for developing health promotion interventions and not the means of evaluating their effect.

- Outcomes occur on a continuum; a focus on proximal indicators is all that is required where we already have evidence for a relationship between indicators and distal outcomes.

- To design our evaluation we must ask how the evaluation will be used and work backwards from this question.

- Even in resource-poor settings, small-scale documentation of the process can contribute to the incremental growth of the evidence base.

References

Andreasen, A.R. (1985) Backward market research. *Harvard Business Review May/June*, 176–82.

Briss, P.A., Zaza, S., Pappaioanou, M. *et al.* (2000) Developing an evidence-based Guide to Community Preventive Services – Methods. The Task Force on Community Preventive Services. *American Journal of Preventive Medicine* **18**(1 Suppl.), 35–43.

Catford, J. (2009) Editorial: Advancing the 'science of delivery' of health promotion: not just the 'science of discovery'. *Health Promotion International* **24**(1),1–5.

Fewtrell, L., Kaufmann, R., Kay, D., Enanonia, W., Haller, L., and Calford, J. (2005) Water, sanitation, and hygiene interventions to reduce diarrhoea in less developed countries: a systematic review and meta-analysis. *Lancet Infectious Diseases* **5**, 42–52.

Green, J. and Tone, K. (1999) Towards a secure evidence base for health promotion. *Journal of Public Health Medicine* **21**(2), 133–9.

Habicht, J.P., Victoria, C.G., and Vaughan, J.P. (1999) Evaluation designs for adequacy, plausibility and probability of public health programme performance and impact. *International Journal of Epidemiology* **28**, 10–18.

Klein, M. and Coombes, Y. (2005) Trust and condom use: the role of sexual caution and sexual assurances for Tanzania youth. *PSI Research Division Working Paper No.* **64**.

McQueen, D.V. (2001) Strengthening the evidence base for health promotion. *Health Promotion International* **16**(3), 261–8.

Nutbeam, D. (1998) Evaluating health promotion – progress, problems and solutions. *Health Promotion International* **13**, 27–43.

Nutbeam, D. (1999) The challenge to provide evidence in health promotion. *Health Promotion International* **14**(2), 99–101.

Raphael, D. (2000) The question of evidence in health promotion. *Health Promotion International* **15**(4), 355–67.

Speller, V., Wimbush, E., and Morgan, A. (2005) Evidence based health promotion practice: how to make it work. *Promotion and Education* Suppl. 1, 15–20.

Tones, K. (1997) Beyond the randomised controlled trial: a case for a judicial review. *Health Education Research* **12**, 1–4.

Chapter 4

Evaluating interventions: experimental study designs in health promotion

Annie Britton

An experimental study is the standard method for evaluating the effectiveness of a health or medical intervention. In such a study, a group of people will be exposed to an intervention and then compared with another group (a control group) who have not been exposed, or with a group who had a different intervention. There are situations in which an experimental approach may not be feasible, ethical, or practical, but, when possible, well-designed controlled experiments provide reliable evidence on the effectiveness of interventions and inform the policies and practice of health promotion.

There is a range of experimental study designs with different advantages and strengths. The findings of randomized controlled trials (RCTs) are perceived as reliable and valid evidence, and are highly valued in clinical research, but their use in health promotion has been criticized (Rosen *et al.* 2006a). There is a suspicion about the perceived dominance of a biomedical system of thought which imposes inappropriate rules, and fails to take account of the complex nature, settings, and long duration of most health promotion interventions. However, a lack of RCT evidence should not be interpreted as a weakness. Well-conducted non-randomized studies, corroborated by other qualitative evidence, can provide a sound evidence base for health promotion interventions.

This chapter discusses the different experimental designs, explores their strengths and weaknesses, and determines how the most appropriate design might be chosen in light of the many unique features of health promotion interventions.

Experimental research

When testing the effectiveness of an intervention we are asking whether the outcome is attributable to the intervention or whether it is a chance occurrence, or perhaps due to some other related factor. This requires a well-planned study with a rigorous design.

The idea of testing the effectiveness of a treatment by experimentation on humans has been around for a long time. One elegant experiment was carried out as early as 1747 by a ship's surgeon who was looking for a cure for the scurvy which was then a major problem for the British Navy, causing more deaths than 'the united efforts of the French and Spanish arms' (Buck *et al.* 1988). James Lind describes how he took 12 sailors with scurvy whose cases were 'as similar as I could get them'. The sailors 'lay together in one place' and had 'one diet common to all'. They were assigned, in pairs, six different medications, including vinegar, cider, sea water, 'elixir vitriol', and 'each two oranges and one lemon every day'. The results were dramatic: 'the most sudden and good effects were perceived from the use of the oranges and lemon; one of those who had taken them being at the end of six days fit for duty'. This early example of a clinical trial contained many of the aspects that are still important in the design of health care trials:

- the question to be addressed had important public health implications;

- more than one treatment was used and the effects were compared (there was a *control group*);

- Lind attempted to choose patients who were similar and to treat them similarly in all other ways except for the treatment being compared in order to eliminate the effect of other factors, such as severity of disease that might otherwise have affected the result; that is, he tried to match the groups for *confounding factors*.

We do not know whether Lind allocated the treatments randomly, but apart from that, this scientific experiment had many features required in a clinical trial today.

Hierarchy of evidence

There are different experimental study designs to choose from with a perceived hierarchy of reliability (see Box 4.1). The results of RCTs

Box 4.1 Hierarchy of experimental research evidence

1. Meta-analysis of high-quality RCTs
2. Single well-designed RCT
3. Well-designed controlled study with quasi-randomization
4. Well-designed controlled study with no randomization
5. 'Before and after' study
6. Study with no control group

and their meta-analyses are at the top of the list. This hierarchy is fundamental for evidence-based medicine and is constructed from an assessment of how much the study designs may be affected by bias, and therefore how certain we can be that the observed effects are attributable to the intervention. The value of the evidence also depends on how well the study was designed, conducted, analysed, and reported. Poor-quality RCTs are less useful than well-designed non-randomized studies.

Randomized controlled trials

The two essential features of an RCT are that at least two interventions are compared, and that people are allocated *at random* to the different groups. Randomization is important because it means that any confounding factors, whether or not they had been previously identified, are likely to be distributed equally between the groups. Hence any difference in outcome can be attributed with more certainty to the difference in the interventions, rather than the effect of confounding. Confounding factors are those that are linked to both the intervention and outcome and can therefore distort the estimated effect. For example, common confounding factors are age and sex. A person's age and sex are likely to affect the way they react to an intervention and both are also important risk factors for many health outcomes.

It could be argued that withholding a health promotion initiative from some individuals just so that a randomized trial can be conducted is unethical or unfair. However, this argument is only relevant if the intervention already has a proven benefit and is being tested in a new setting or mode of delivery. Most agree that it is ethical to randomize when it is *uncertain* whether a new intervention is superior to an older one after benefits, risks, and costs have been taken into account. Part of the ethics of RCTs is to have stopping rules for when an intervention is shown to be significantly harmful or beneficial. Moreover, if an intervention is introduced in a 'phased' manner (see Box 4.2) it is possible to conduct an RCT and to enable everyone to eventually receive the intervention (Rosen *et al.* 2006b).

The unit of randomization can be either an individual person or a group of people, for example a family, school, medical practice, or even a whole town. The latter kind of randomization is particularly useful when a community-based intervention is being tested. Such trials are called *cluster randomized trial*s and an example is described in Box 4.2.

It is important that neither the researcher who is allocating the intervention groups, nor the participant who is being allocated to a

Box 4.2 Randomized controlled trial of preschool hand-washing initiative

Researchers in Jerusalem wanted to test whether a hygiene health promotion programme in preschools could reduce the incidence of upper-respiratory-tract infection. Forty preschools (involving 1029 children) were randomized to either an intervention or a control group. The programme used a multi-pronged approach that included elements aimed at staff, children, parents, school nurses, and changes to the classroom environment. An approximately threefold increase in hand washing with soap was observed among preschool children exposed to the intervention. However, there was no reduction in absenteeism due to illness. Shortly after, the programme was implemented in the control preschools, thus ensuring that eventually all the children received the programme in a 'phased' manner (Rosen *et al.* 2006b).

group, can predict or influence the allocation. This is called *concealed allocation* and is done to prevent any possibility of bias arising from either the participant or the researcher preferring one intervention to another. It is also preferable, if possible, that neither the researchers nor the participants in the study are aware who is receiving which intervention during the trial so that compliance to the study and measurement of the outcome cannot be affected. This is called *double-blinding*. Such trials are relatively easy to conduct when the treatment is a pill for which an inactive but otherwise identical placebo can be prepared. It is much less easy in trials of health promotion interventions.

Systematic reviews and meta-analyses can be used to assess the quality and combine the evidence from many different RCTs. They are discussed fully in Chapter 6.

Unique features of health promotion

Rigorous evaluation is important, but that does not mean that an RCT is the best method in every circumstance. The aims of health promotion differ in important ways from those of the curative interventions. There are two dimensions of health promotion that should be considered in planning or reviewing experimental studies that evaluate health promotion interventions: the nature of the intervention and the nature of the participants.

Nature of the intervention

The intervention being tested in a clinical trial usually has a biological basis (for example, drugs, surgery, or physiotherapy). In health promotion, interventions rarely involve direct manipulation of the biological environment. Health promotion interventions aim to achieve behavioural change at either an individual or a societal level. This has repercussions for the design of trials, both in terms of the unit that receives the intervention (which could be an individual, a family, a small community, or a whole nation, for example), and in terms of the concepts of placebo comparisons and blinding. It is difficult to devise a placebo comparison for a community-development intervention, and almost always impossible to blind people to the fact that that they have received a health promotion initiative such as counselling or group therapy.

Often the goal of health promotion interventions is to prevent ill health a long way in the future. For example, a community project which was concerned with improving access to fresh fruit and vegetables would be expected to impact the health of the population over a period of many years, as children grew up with a more adequate intake of antioxidants. The focus of health promotion on outcomes in the distant future makes evaluation by RCTs difficult and expensive. However, even if the outcome is long-term, we can look at changes in behaviour, or even intention-to-change measures as proximal indicators of the outcome measure (see Chapter 3 for a discussion on the relationship between proximal and outcome indicators). Not all health promotion is long-term; for example, interventions that prevent communicable diseases may have measurable effects quickly.

When a community-level intervention is being evaluated there is a risk that neighbouring communities that are acting as control groups will adopt the practices of the intervention community. After all, health promotion interventions address important health problems and it is likely that many communities are looking for solutions to the same problems. This *contamination* is hard to prevent and control.

Nature of the participants

In a health promotion trial, the participants are unlikely to be seeking a solution for their health problem: in fact, it is possible that the subjects do not perceive that they have a health problem. Clinical trials aim to find a way to cure or ameliorate a condition, and in such trials the participants enter the trial with a health problem from which they hope to find relief. Often, people will describe their motivation for entering such a trial as 'to help find a cure'. This will not be the case in a health promotion RCT but there may be other motivations for people joining the trial (for example, support to exercise or diet) and this will affect recruitment to a trial. The problem of biased recruitment is discussed in the next section.

Validity of trials

Internal and external validity are both important when evaluating the importance of trial findings. *The internal validity* is a measure of the extent to which the findings are real and not the result of bias. The groups that are compared should be as alike as possible, except for the intervention under investigation. In well-conducted, blinded, RCTs internal validity is not usually a problem.

When a trial is not blinded and the participants are aware of their allocation, results could be biased by the effects of participant preferences. Participants often have strong preferences or beliefs about the effectiveness of interventions and this may enhance or reduce their response (possibly through compliance or via psychological pathways). In a trial of smoking-cessation interventions, for example, participants may receive either counselling for smoking cessation or hypnosis therapy. If an individual has a strong belief in the effectiveness of hypnosis, they may experience an enhanced response if randomized to the hypnosis arm of the trial, and a more negative effect if randomized to counselling. It is very difficult to measure the consequences of preference effects (McPherson 2009), but researchers need to be aware of them when planning trials.

External validity is a measure of how generalizable the findings are to the wider population. Individuals who participate in health promotion trials are more likely to be younger, to be of higher socio-economic status, and to have a healthier lifestyle in comparison to non-participants (Britton *et al.* 1998). Where participants are found to differ from the rest of the population, the external validity of the study is weakened.

The external validity can also be compromised by the conditions in which a trial is conducted, which are sometimes far removed from real-life practice. When the eligibility criteria are very strict and 100% compliance is achieved, such trials are called efficacy trials because they measure the extent to which a specific intervention, procedure or service produces a beneficial result under ideal conditions. Such findings may not be generalizable or repeatable in normal practice. An effectiveness or pragmatic trial is one which takes place in a normal practice setting and is therefore subject to the hazards of non-compliance and loss to follow-up. The participants may be very heterogeneous and have co-morbidities, but therefore such trials have higher external validity.

The importance of external validity has increased with the need to understand how research findings can be translated to public health practice. To assess external validity and decide whether a trial's impact can be replicated in other settings, researchers should report on methodological issues such as recruitment and selection procedures, participation rates, consistency of implementation across programme components, and attrition at all levels (Steckler and McLeroy 2008).

Complex interventions

Health promotion initiatives often require complex interventions, characterized by several interacting components, involvement of many groups or organizational levels and a number of different outcomes. An example of a highly complex intervention is Sure Start. Launched in 1998, Sure Start is a UK Government initiative with the aim of 'giving children the best possible start in life' through improvement of childcare, early education, health, and family support, with an emphasis on outreach and community development (Box 4.3).

Box 4.3 Example of a non-randomised study

Sure Start Local Programmes (SSLPs) are area-based interventions to improve services for young children and their families in deprived communities in England, promote health and development, and reduce inequalities. To evaluate the effectiveness of the programmes a comparison was made of the wellbeing of 3-year-old children and their families in a sample of 93 SSLP areas and in 72 similarly deprived non-SSLP areas in England.

After controlling for pre-existing background differences of children, families, areas, and time of measurement (possible confounding factors), the researchers found beneficial effects associated with the programme for five of 14 outcomes (better social development, better behaviour, greater independence, less-negative parenting, and better home-learning environment) (Melhuish *et al.* 2008).

In 2000, the UK Medical Research Council published a framework to help researchers to recognize and adopt appropriate methods. This guidance has recently been revised and updated (<http://www.mrc.ac.uk/complexinterventionsguidance>). While recognizing that RCTs provide reliable evaluation evidence, the new framework recommends consideration of alternative study designs and emphasizes contextual considerations (Craig *et al.* 2008).

Alternative forms of experimental evaluation

Studies with a current comparison group but without randomization (quasi-randomized or non-randomized studies)

Where it is unethical or impractical to allocate people randomly to interventions, it may be possible to conduct a study using a quasi-randomized method, for example allocating by order of presentation (see Box 4.4) or first letter of surname. These methods attempt to limit selection bias although it is possible that participants may manipulate the allocation method in order to be assigned to their preferred experimental group.

Non-randomized studies are those in which the investigator or participants choose their intervention or are allocated on some other

---

Box 4.4 Example of a quasi-randomized study

To test whether yoga in the third trimester will improve pregnancy and childbirth among first-time mothers, researchers recruited women attending a prenatal clinic in Taiwan. The first 43 women were given usual care (control group) and the next 45 were given a 12-week yoga programme consisting of a booklet, video tape, and follow-up telephone calls. Comparisons were made to check there were no differences in terms of maternal and newborn characteristics between the control and experimental groups. Women who took part in the prenatal yoga programme reported significantly fewer pregnancy discomforts at 38–40 weeks' gestation and better labour experience than the control group (Sun *et al.* 2009).

basis, for example geographical location (see Box 4.3). When the investigator or participant chooses the allocation, the study groups may differ with respect to confounding factors (age, sex, socio-economic status, and other risk factors that affect outcome), which makes it difficult to ascertain the intervention effect. Such studies should only be considered where RCTs are not possible. There is always a risk that any difference in outcome between non-randomized groups is due to some unmeasured confounding factor and the effectiveness of the health promotion initiative under investigation is measured with imprecision. All important characteristics of the two groups should be measured before the trial starts so that stratification and statistical adjustments can be made in the analyses.

Studies with no current comparison group

Sometimes it is not possible to find an appropriate comparison group. This is usually because the intervention being evaluated has extended over a whole population. In this case the best alternative may be for the intervention group to act as their own control, so that the effect of the intervention is estimated from the observed change over the period of the intervention. This is sometimes described as a *before-and-after study* (Box 4.5). These studies have many weaknesses, particularly as they cannot eliminate the effects of any other changes that occur over time. However, they can sometimes provide the only available evidence of whether or not an intervention was effective.

Box 4.5 Example of a before-and-after study

Between 1989 and 1991 in Thailand a rapid increase in the prevalence of HIV infection in female sex workers was noted, from 3.5 to 15% prevalence. In response, the Ministry of Public Health set up the '100% Condom Campaign' to control the spread of infection. This was a national campaign, so no current control group was available. The initiative was evaluated by a study of a series of five cohorts of army recruits between 1991 and 1995. Between 1991 and 1993 the prevalence of HIV in army recruits ranged between 10 and 13%. By 1995, it had fallen to 7% (Nelson *et al.* 1996).

Box 4.6 Questions to ask when designing a research study

All study designs should address the following questions.

1. Is your study group representative of the wider population of interest?

2. Is your sample size large enough to detect a statistically significant intervention effect?

3. How will you deal with people who do not comply with the study protocol or who are lost at follow-up?

4. Will useful evidence come from a qualitative evaluation conducted alongside the quantitative evaluation?

If an RCT has been chosen, think about these questions.

1. What is the most efficient unit of randomization (individual or cluster)?

2. Is it possible to blind the trial participants to the allocation of the intervention and control?

3. Is it possible to blind the people measuring the outcome to the allocation of the intervention and control?

4. At what stage of the study will randomization occur?

If a non-RCT has been chosen, think about these questions.

1. Are the intervention and control groups similar for known confounders?

2. Can known confounders be measured at baseline and adjusted for in the analyses?

If a study with no current comparison group is chosen, think about these questions.

1. Are there any identifiable time trends (apart from the planned intervention) which are likely to distort the results? Can these be measured and adjusted for?

2. Is it possible to identify a sample (of individuals or communities) that can be studied at baseline and then at points during and after the intervention?

3. If not, how will the expected change in the population be measured?

Conflicting evidence from different study designs

There are a number of instances where a widespread practice has been challenged by conflicting evidence from health promotion studies. For example, there was evidence from many non-randomized studies that using hormone-replacement therapy halves the risk of coronary heart disease. However, the pooled results from three randomized trials did not show this apparent cardioprotective effect (Beral *et al.* 2002). In this case it is likely that the results from the non-randomized studies are erroneous because of residual confounding; that is, women who take hormone-replacement therapy smoke less, take more exercise, and are more affluent than women who do not use hormone-replacement therapy.

Similarly, although non-randomized studies suggested a preventive effect of β-carotene and vitamin A on lung cancer and cardiovascular disease, a controlled trial was stopped early due to interim results that showed a possible adverse effect on those endpoints (Omenn *et al.* 1996). Again, residual confounding in the non-randomized studies is likely to explain the discrepancy. These examples serve as a reminder of how we need to be cautious when interpreting the results of non-randomized studies (Lawlor *et al.* 2004).

Choosing an appropriate study design

When conducting research, particularly within the field of health promotion evaluation, the choice of whether to use a randomized or non-randomized strategy will be dictated by practicalities. Box 4.6 illustrates the basic questions to be addressed at the design stage. Once a method of evaluation has been chosen, the work is only just beginning. The challenge is to design and carry out the most reliable and valid study possible.

Key points

♦ Well-conducted RCTs are a valid and important way of evaluating health promotion interventions.

♦ RCTs are not always appropriate or feasible and other forms of evaluation must be used.

♦ RCTs are useful for measuring the effects of interventions but not for explaining why these effects occur.

♦ Researchers should report on the external validity of trial findings to assist translation of research into public health practice.

References

Beral, V., Banks, F., Reeves, G. (2002) Evidence from randomized trials on the long-term effects of hormone replacement therapy. *Lancet* **360**, 942–4.

Britton, A.R., Mckee, M., Black, N., McPherson, K., Sanderson, C., and Bain, C. (1998) Choosing between randomized and non-randomized studies. A systematic review. *Health Technology Assessment* **2**(13), 1–124.

Buck, C., Llopis, A., Najera, E., and Terris, M. (1988) *The Challenge of Epidemiology: Issues and Selected Readings.* Pan American Health Organizations, Washington DC.

Craig, P., Dieppe, P., Macintyre, S., Mitchie, S., Nazareth, I., and Petticrew, M. (2008) Developing and evaluating complex interventions: the new Medical Research Council guidance. *British Medical Journal* **337**, 979–83.

Lawlor, D.A., Davey Smith, G., Bruckdorfer, K.R., Kundu, D., and Ebrahim, S. (2004) Those confounded vitamins: what can we learn from the differences between observational versus randomised trial evidence? *Lancet* **363**, 1724–7.

McPherson, K. (2009) Do patients' preferences matter? *British Medical Journal* **338**, 59–60.

Melhuish, E., Belsky, J., Leyland, A.H., and Barnes, J. (2008). Effects of fully-established Sure Start Local Programmes on 3-year-old children and their families living in England: a quasi-experimental observational study. *Lancet* **372**, 1641–7.

Nelson, K.E., Celentano, D.D., Eiumtrakol, S. *et al.* (1996) Changes in sexual behaviour and a decline in HIV infection among young men in Thailand. *New England Journal of Medicine* **355**, 297–303.

Omenn, G., Goodman, G., Thornquist, D. *et al.* (1996) Effects of a combination of beta carotene and vitamin A on lung cancer and cardiovascular disease. *New England Journal of Medicine* **334**, 1150–5.

Rosen, L., Manor, O., Engelhard, D., and Zucker, D. (2006a) In defence of the randomized controlled trial for health promotion research. *American Journal of Public Health* **96**, 1181–6.

Rosen, L., Manor, O., Engelhard, D. *et al.* (2006b) Can a handwashing intervention make a difference? Results from a randomised controlled trial in Jerusalem preschools. *Preventive Medicine* **42**, 27–32.

Steckler, A. and McLeroy, K.R. (2008). The importance of external validity. *American Journal of Public Health* **98**, 9–10.

Sun, Y., Hung, Yi., Chang, Y., and Kuo, S. (2009) Effects of a prenatal yoga programme on the discomforts of pregnancy and maternal childbirth self-efficacy in Taiwan. *Midwifery* (in press).

Chapter 5

Economic evaluation of health promotion interventions

Warren Stevens

Economic evaluation in health care is often misrepresented; it is seen as an attempt by economists to put a price on a life. This is an over-simplification of the theory, but does act as a useful starting point for an explanation of its value to decision-makers and health promotion researchers. Every time we use scarce resources in one area, we leave other areas with fewer available resources as a result. As the poor person of health care, health promotion has the most to gain from garnering evidence of its value relative to the traditionally more heavily funded areas of investment such as therapeutic interventions. For health promotion, economic evaluation has the potential to be both a research and important advocacy tool.

Economic evaluation can show health promotion interventions in their true light; as a valuable source of investment in health in comparison with traditional health care. Parameters such as cost per life year saved or cost per infection averted are already becoming more widely accepted in all areas of health research. Hybrid measures of health outcomes such as quality-adjusted life years or disability-adjusted life years, that combine either quality of life or morbidity with mortality, are gaining greater support by both researchers and decision-makers. All health interventions are an investment in future health and wellbeing; the use of economic evaluation has the power to show where and when intervening early can have a better return than curative approaches requiring clinical intervention. In a world where equity is developing into a significant goal for all health systems, intervening earlier avoids the ever-increasing health inequalities associated with the utilization of health care.

This chapter touches on the theory behind finite resources, the need for systems of allocation, and the value of optimization of benefits within limited resources. It then goes on to look more practically at the major issues that are encountered when measuring costs and benefits, dealing with uncertainty and the difficulties that surround transferring results from one location to another. Finally there is a cost-effectiveness case study of a malaria-prevention intervention in Malawi, and a discussion that takes us through some of the more common debates in the field.

Theory into practice

Welfare economics proposes that when all individuals maximize their health outcomes then society as a whole has maximized its health outcomes. Given a world of finite resources, the aim to maximize health outcomes is only restricted by the resources we have to achieve this goal. So, the cheaper and more beneficial each health care intervention is, the more likely it is to move us towards our society's goal of health maximization. We therefore need to know how much benefit each intervention can give us for each dollar we invest, so that we allocate our resources such that our health benefits are maximized.

Economics looks at how best to allocate limited resources to satisfy often-unlimited demand. All resources are limited; no matter how much there is of something, it will eventually run out. Economists attempt to maximize aggregate benefit from within the restriction of limited resources. The theory of benefit maximization is best described in terms of Pareto efficiency.

Pareto efficiency was named after the economist Vilfredo Pareto. He stated that any redistribution of resources would improve efficiency if it made at least one person better off without making anyone else worse off. Society would therefore be most efficient where it is impossible to redistribute resources to make someone better off without simultaneously making someone else worse off. There could be a number of different permutations of resource allocation that resulted in Pareto efficiency, but they would all produce the exact same level of aggregate benefit. This is perfectly acceptable in theory but becomes difficult to measure in practice. For example, how is benefit defined? Do some things benefit some people more than others?

The concept has been further developed by the compensation principle introduced by Kaldor and Hicks in 1939, which adds the concept of relative or net benefit, making the model more flexible. If a redistribution of resources results in gainers and losers, it is a move towards Pareto efficiency but only if the aggregate benefits of the gainers outweigh the aggregate costs of the losers. In principle the gainers can then compensate the losers while still achieving a net benefit. Kaldor and Hicks proposed that the measurement of benefit should be directly comparable with the costs of redistribution and should be given a monetary value.

Thus, from welfare economics with the goal of optimizing the distribution of scarce resources combined with the tenets of the theories of *allocative* efficiency, we reach the theoretical base for the development of the economic evaluation of public services. This being that, it is not possible to decide the resource allocation of public services by the market due to the market's imperfect nature (this would require all 'users' of health care to have perfect information about the product). The allocation of resources, therefore, requires some form of intervention by government, if the goal is to maximize the health of the entire population. These resources need to be directed by a definitive measurement of all alternative methods of health investment. One such method is the quantification of each health care intervention in terms of its return on investment, expressed as the health benefits accrued for each dollar spent.

General concepts

Having agreed that society's goal is welfare maximization, through funding directed towards the most cost-effective interventions, we now have to address the more practical issue of measurement. Cost-effectiveness is a simple concept in theory: measuring the benefits from a chosen intervention against the costs borne by undertaking it. However, this simple concept must take place in a complex world, where there are many contextual factors that will impact on both the outcomes and costs of an intervention. More often than not 'complete' measurement of the costs and benefits of an intervention is impossible, and what has emerged is a science that measures cost-effectiveness in graduations, based in part on the degree to which it is practical to measure them.

Cost-effectiveness is often used as a catchall phrase but is simultaneously one of four variations on the same theme. At one time or another you will hear of cost-benefit, cost-utility, or cost-minimization (sometimes called cost-neutral) analyses, as well as the better-known cost-effectiveness. These terms differ only by how they measure outcomes, and to what purpose.

The roots of the economic evaluation method is cost-benefit analysis, the aim of which is to measure the effect of changes in resource allocation in terms of the net benefit to society. It differs from the more commonly referenced cost-effectiveness analyses in the sense that benefits are measured in terms of money. The original purpose of cost-benefit analyses was to measure whether the value accrued in the long term outweighed the initial investment. Cost-benefit analyses, although popular in other areas of social investment such as road building and housing, is rarely used in health care due to the complex nature of measuring health outcomes. A version of cost-effectiveness analysis, known as cost-utility analysis (CUA) attempts to overcome this problem by using a common measure of outcome, so the relative cost-effectiveness of all interventions can be compared. In CUA the benefits are expressed in terms of quality-adjusted life years (QALYs), disability-adjusted life years (DALYs), or the more recent healthy-year-equivalents (HYEs). These CUA methods can then be used to compare interventions with different outcomes.

CUA continues to be the fastest growing form of economic evaluation, although there is ongoing debate about the use and calculation of each of the hybrid measures of benefit. The application of these methods is under continuous review, with no consensus of opinion (Drummond *et al.* 2001). The choice of method is not always straightforward. Options may be limited due to the type and quality of the data available, as well as constraints on time and resources. When deciding on a methodology and an outcome measure the goal must be to maximize what can be achieved and to choose the method most appropriate to the data.

Measuring cost and effectiveness

Nothing exists within an academic discipline without some level of debate, and measuring true economic cost is no exception. The three major areas of debate in cost measurement are:

◆ the *perspective* from which our measure of cost originates;

◆ inter-temporal differences in real cost, or *discounting*; and

◆ international differences in purchasing power, or *shadow pricing*.

Perspective

There are two broad areas of perspective, known as the provider and societal perspectives. The *provider perspective* is a supply-side measure, used where evaluation results are destined for a specific customer, usually the organization that will need to free up current resources to fund the new intervention. Their objectives are to understand what costs the provider will have to bear, what potential savings the provider could make, and what improvements in overall health benefit will be gained by the population that the provider serves.

Alternatively a study measured from a *societal perspective* must go outside the impact of the immediate provider and attempt to capture all relevant costs that are borne by providers, potential beneficiaries, their families, and other co-existing providers. Thus, all relevant costs and benefits that may accrue across society as a whole are aggregated. These are often termed 'indirect costs'. This method sticks most closely to the ethos of welfare economics; to assess the true benefit to society all benefits and costs should be included. Inevitably, as we move closer to theoretical perfection we are hit harder by practical limitations.

Discounting

The theoretical basis of discounting relates to the fact that costs and benefits have a higher value now than in the future, and so future costs and benefits must be discounted to be compared like for like with those in the present. Intuitively, the opportunity to take any benefit now is preferred to receiving that benefit in the future; similarly the preference is for any costs to be borne in years to come rather than now. This is why we pay such high rates of interest on our mortgages, as we are paying for the right to put off costs until the future. Similarly we receive interest on savings as a reward for not spending the money in the present.

There is much debate in the literature on the necessity and exact value that should be used to discount both costs and benefits (Gravelle and Smith 2001), and when and where they should be used (Walker and Kumaranayake 2002). This is an important point in the evaluation of health promotion investments, as the bulk of benefits will be accrued in the future, whereas the costs are often borne in the present. If the discount rate is too high this will have a significant effect on the perceived value of the intervention compared to interventions where the investment and the health benefits returned both happen in the present.

Shadow pricing

Finally we have the issue of differences in international purchasing power. Shadow pricing is the use of world market or 'border' prices of goods or services used as inputs into the intervention, rather than local prices that may be artificially low or high. The reason for this is partly for translation across borders, but more importantly it is based on the principle of 'opportunity cost', which is the key principle that defines all costs in economic theory.

For example, if a particular good required for an intervention were locally priced much lower than the world market price, a better use of that resource would be to export it onto the world market and gain additional resources to produce more. So instead of handing out 10 locally made bed nets that cost $1 each, if the world market price is $5, exporting the ten bed nets would provide resources for 50 bed nets. In reality perfectly competitive markets tend to prevent these situations from occurring but the prevalence of tariffs and subsidies across borders mean that shadow prices often occur, and to use local prices would be to under- or overestimate true costs drastically. A good review of the issues and methods can be seen in Dinwiddy and Teal (1996).

Generalization and transferability of results

The gold standard for generating robust and acceptable evidence in health interventions is the randomized controlled trial, and for many public health interventions this will be a community-randomized trial. Randomized trials are discussed in Chapter 4, where the issues of internal and external validity are described.

As part of achieving internal validity a series of exclusions and restrictions will be put on entrants to the trial. Any differences in relative risk, age, and background are effectively lost, as are factors that could affect the outcome one way or the other, such as co-morbidities or poor adherence. As a result any difference between the two groups is a difference only relevant to those types of people and communities not excluded from the study. Studies have shown that such criteria can exclude an important proportion of the population these interventions will eventually be aimed at (Travers *et al.* 2007, Van Spall *et al.* 2007).

Another problem with the generalizability of evidence derived from the experimental method is the importance placed on internal validity. The goal of the controlled trial is to show that *only* the intervention is responsible for a particular outcome. But this can mask why a specific outcome was achieved (the process of the intervention; see Chapter 7 for a more thorough discussion of process evaluation). The fact that the existence of contextual differences that impact on the relative success of an intervention are rarely recorded or reported when reporting such studies has been highlighted as a major barrier to the acceptance of evidence in policy decisions (Cronbach 1993).

A further component of trial design that leads to the potential loss of valuable contextual data is the desire for a trial to generate statistically significant results. A by-product of this is that statistical significance is determined by sample size and as such most trials pool all available data to generate an overall difference of effect. As a result, potentially valuable information on specific subgroups within the population is lost. In fact the analysis of such data across subgroups is often unfairly frowned on, despite the acknowledgement that heterogeneity of effect within populations exists, and that such heterogeneity may be a significant cause of variance in terms of an intervention's overall effectiveness across a population (Birch *et al.* 2007).

The process of translating evidence into valuable and quantifiable information that can direct interventions and programme implementation is one that requires attention by the research community;

indeed, it has recently generated a whole new area of study (Eccles and Mittman 2006). The importance of the process of translating evidence should be considered as one of the key components in trial design. If we are going to direct research towards having accountability as to the value of the results it produces, then designing studies and collecting data that is integral to the use of these results in directing policy is as important, if not more important, than the summary statistics that traditionally describe the effectiveness of the interventions.

Reporting uncertainty

Economic evaluation has been accused of lacking scientific rigour compared to the methods pursued in controlled trials. Initially cost-effectiveness was measured deterministically (point estimates of cost and effect), but most economic evaluations nowadays measure cost-effectiveness using stochastic methods (Briggs *et al.* 1999) to allow the presentation of results alongside more traditional statistical measures of uncertainty such as confidence intervals. As cost-effectiveness is not a single measure but a ratio of two measures—costs and effect— this has led to the development of new sets of tools for reporting results such as cost-efficacy spheres, ellipses, or ovals. These are not more complex measures of cost-effectiveness but simply variations in the way the data is presented, and they allow for a more open approach to the reporting of the data.

Efficiency versus equality: a trade-off?

In both theoretical and applied welfare economics there is the concept of an efficiency/equality trade-off: that greater overall level of efficiency in health care delivery cannot be achieved without some loss to certain groups within the population. For example, immunization programmes with the aim of maximizing coverage often leave the poorest children un-immunized. The trade-off discussion began in macroeconomics, but the concept has now been incorporated in more specific areas of welfare economics, including health care (Bosanquet 2001).

Elsewhere initiatives are being introduced and tested to assess the economic viability of targeting the very poor in public health programmes by paying people to attend or to comply with programmes

(Morris *et al.* 2004). These programmes have shown that it is economically viable to pay certain groups to attend nominally free public health interventions that they were not previously utilizing. The benefits gained by society as a whole are likely to be greater than the costs incurred in providing the incentive. This contradicts the theory that maximizing benefits and reducing inequalities cannot be achieved simultaneously.

So why is a previously intractable problem being turned on its head? The key to understanding how targeting reductions in inequality can be a means of increasing efficiency is in dissecting the definition and measurement of both attributes.

Traditionally the relationship between efficiency and equality has been structured as inverse. An $x\%$ increase in efficiency would mean a $y\%$ decrease in equality. For example, it is widely accepted that the poor are the last to be reached when immunization programmes are scaled up. It is also generally accepted that to increase coverage in targeted areas has additional costs that drive an upward sloping cost curve. This means to get an immunization coverage rate of 50% costs about $\$a$ per person covered, whereas to increase that coverage rate to 60% would mean a cost per person covered of $\$(a+n)$, for 70% $\$(a+2n)$, and so on.

This argument relies very much on the assumption of a homogenous population, where potential health outcomes from universal health interventions are spread evenly across the population. Studies that look at the relationship between health and social inequalities tell us this is not the case. The use of average 'impact' for an intervention then fails to allow for the importance of the heterogeneity within populations in the capacity to benefit from health interventions.

Traditionally we see the cost-effectiveness of health interventions as having a U-shaped cost curve; initially economies of scale are achieved but as coverage grows the diseconomies associated with striving to achieve coverage in the more difficult sections of the population are realized, and unit costs rise as a result. What is not always incorporated into these studies is the level of heterogeneity in the benefits gained per person as coverage rises, and those whose burden of disease is higher start to be covered. If it is true that as coverage increases

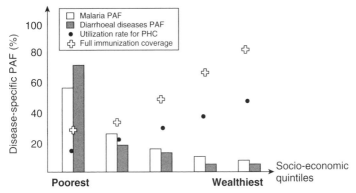

Fig. 5.1 Population-attributable risk and utilization/coverage rates by socio-economic quintile

PAF, population-attributable fraction; PHC, primary health care.

Sources: Ezzati *et al.* (2003), Gwatkin *et al.* (2004).

average costs can rise, it is also true that as coverage rises so average benefit increases.

This argument relies heavily on two assumptions. The first is that those least likely to benefit from a health intervention are those most likely to receive it. Assumption number two is that this effect is measurable and therefore quantifiable. The first can be addressed through any number of studies that look at the relationship between social or economic status and utilization of health services (see Figure 5.1).

The second assumption is more difficult to address, as it is more subjective. What constitutes a 'measurable' variance between groups? Measurability of effect between groups is no more difficult to measure than across an entire population, if the same rules are applied to both questions (Stevens and Normand 2004). The choice of whether to pursue these goals simultaneously is still guided in part by evidence but also in part by philosophy, but the issue of inequalities in health and its role in the evaluation of heath interventions cannot be ignored.

A cost-effectiveness case study of a malaria-prevention intervention in Malawi is presented in Box 5.1.

Box 5.1 Case study. Cost-effectiveness of delivering insecticide-treated nets in Malawi

Background

Between 1998 and 2003 the Malawian government, Population Services International (an international non-governmental organization), and a series of donors (including the United States Agency for International Development, the UK Department for International Development) implemented a social marketing insecticide-treated net (ITN) programme across Malawi. The strategy involved segmenting the market such that a full-cost net was made available to all consumers and a subsidized net was made available to pregnant women and children under 5 (those most at risk of death from malaria) through public health facilities. The nets were heavily promoted to the public through a range of mass-media and interpersonal communications channels.

Methods

A cost-effectiveness study, with measures including cost per life saved, was used to make the results comparable both with other malaria interventions and with other health interventions on a wider scale. Costs were broken down into capital costs, which were annualized and discounted across their life span, and recurrent or programme costs. The latter were broken down into direct costs, and shared costs. An appropriate apportionment method was chosen for each type of expenditure. Capital items were annualized over assumed life spans, in line with comparable studies. The discount rate used was 3%, and costs were measured in a combination of local currency (Malawi Kwacha) and in US dollars, depending on whether the resources were purchased or paid locally or overseas. All costs were then translated into US dollars. Outcomes were estimated by combining numbers of ITN distributed, coverage and utilization data from surveillance studies, and efficacy data from systematic reviews. When combined using probabilistic modelling these produced a series of deaths averted and DALY averted outcomes.

Box 5.1 Case study. Cost-effectiveness of delivering insecticide-treated nets in Malawi *(cont)*

Results

The average economic cost per death averted and the average cost per DALY averted, over the 5 years, were $1105–22 and $30–7 respectively. The interesting aspect of this study is the gains from cost savings that are accrued from distribution of ITN at a larger scale, or what is often termed scale efficiency savings. Here the cost per DALY averted dropped from $52 to $24 as annual ITNs delivered rose from 72 196 to 720 577.

Discussion

The goal for economists and policy-makers is to determine the method, or combinations of methods, that can ensure the best way of achieving a sustainable high level of utilization of this product in communities where the benefits are highest. This study suggests that a combination of building local markets, and targeting vulnerable groups, could achieve relatively high levels of coverage over time with proper investment. In addition it may be possible to achieve high levels of ITN coverage while keeping unit costs down by achieving increasing returns to scale (Stevens *et al.* 2005).

Key points

- ◆ Resources are not infinite so decisions must be made as to how resources should best be allocated to maximize health benefits.
- ◆ Economic evaluation can be a powerful tool in comparing the value of health promotion interventions with more traditional therapeutic interventions.
- ◆ Choosing the type of economic evaluation relies on understanding the perspective; the comparison to be made, and the data that are likely to be available.

- ◆ The key to maximizing the potential transferability of findings is transparency of both methods and results, the intrinsic incorporation of context, and generous use of sensitivity analysis.

- ◆ Efficiency and equity are two equally admirable goals, and they can be achieved without compromise to each other.

References

Birch, S., Haas, M., Savage, E., and Van Gool, K. (2007) Targeting services to reduce social inequalities in utilisation: an analysis of breast cancer screening in New South Wales. *Australia and New Zealand Health Policy* **4**, 12

Bosanquet, N. (2001) A 'fair innings' for efficiency in health services? *Journal of Medical Ethics* **27**(4), 228–33.

Briggs, A.H., Mooney, C.Z., and Wonderling, D.E. (1999) Constructing confidence intervals for cost-effectiveness ratios: an evaluation of parametric and non-parametric techniques using Monte Carlo simulation. *Statistics in Medicine* **18**(23), 3245–62.

Cronbach, L. (1993) *Designing Evaluations for Educational and Social Programs.* Jossey-Bass Publications, San Francisco, CA.

Dinwiddy, C. and Teal, F. (1996) *Principles of Cost–Benefit Analysis in Developing Countries.* Cambridge University Press, Cambridge.

Drummond, M., Briggs, A., and McGuire, A. (2001) *Economic Evaluation in Health Care: Merging Theory with Practice.* Oxford University Press, Oxford.

Eccles, M.P. and Mittman, B.S. (2006) Introducing a new field of science. *Implementation Science* **1**, 1.

Ezzati, M., Hoorn, S.V., Rodgers, A., Lopez, A.D., Mathers, C.D., and Murray, C.J. (2003) Comparative Risk Assessment Collaborating Group. Estimates of global and regional potential health gains from reducing multiple major risk factors. *Lancet* **362**(9380), 271–80.

Gravelle, H. and Smith, D. (2001) Discounting for health effects in cost–benefit and cost–effectiveness analysis. *Health Economics* **10**(7), 587–99.

Gwatkin, D.R., Bhuiya, A., and Victora, C.G. (2004) Making health systems more equitable. *Lancet* **364**(9441), 1273–80.

Morris, S.S., Flores, R., Olinto, P., and Medina, J.M. (2004) Monetary incentives in primary health care and effects on use and coverage of preventive health care interventions in rural Honduras: cluster randomised trial. *Lancet* **364**(9450), 2030–7.

Stevens, W. and Normand, C. (2004) Optimisation versus certainty: understanding the issue of heterogeneity in economic evaluation. *Social Science and Medicine* **58**(2), 315–20.

Stevens, W., Wiseman, V., Ortiz, J., and Chavasse, D. (2005) The costs and effects of a nationwide insecticide-treated net programme: the case of Malawi. *Malaria Journal* **4**(1), 22.

Travers, J., Marsh, S., Williams, M. *et al.* (2007) External validity of randomized controlled trials in asthma: to whom do the results of the trials apply? *Thorax* **62**, 219–23.

Van Spall, H.G.C., Toren, A., Kiss, A., and Fowler, R.A. (2007) Eligibility criteria of randomized controlled trials published in high-impact general medical journals. *Journal of the American Medical Association* **297**, 1233–40.

Walker, D. and Kumaranayake, L. (2002) Allowing for differential timing in cost analyses: discounting and annualization. *Health Policy and Planning* **17**(1), 112–18.

Chapter 6

Using systematic reviews in health promotion

Margaret Thorogood

If evidence is to be useful it must be accessible to the people who need it. A policy-maker or practitioner who wanted to know whether a particular activity was effective would be faced with a difficult task in accessing and evaluating all the different evidence. Moreover, the findings of individual intervention studies are sometimes contradictory or the individual studies are too small to provide significant findings and it is only when available research studies are compared *systematically*, or, in the case of meta-analyses, combined, that an estimate of the true effect of an intervention will emerge. A systematic review aims to search for and organize information in a systematic way, using transparent searches and inclusion and exclusion criteria to try, as far as is possible, to provide an unbiased summary of the evidence. Of course, non-systematic reviews by experts exist, and they can be helpful in highlighting the scope of a topic or the range of views, but a systematic review goes further in systematically bringing together all the available evidence.

The idea of systematically bringing together evidence on a topic is not new, but the modern enthusiasm for such reviews can, in large part, be attributed to the influence of one man, Archie Cochrane, who was one of the most influential epidemiologists of the twentieth century. He recognized that most health care interventions had not been evaluated, and many of them might be either ineffectual or harmful. It was his call for the use of critical summaries of randomized controlled trials (RCTs) to evaluate health care interventions that inspired the foundation of the Cochrane Collaboration (The Cochrane Library), which is described below.

This chapter briefly describes how to undertake a systematic review, including the important step of defining the research question, and discusses some of the problems and challenges. Using examples, it describes some of the ways in which systematic reviews can be used in evaluating health promotion, and how to evaluate the quality and relevance of such reviews.

Uses of systematic reviews

Boxes 6.1 to 6.3 show examples of three very different systematic reviews aiming to answer widely different research questions. There are two common ways of reporting systematic reviews: *meta-analyses* and *narrative reviews*. All systematic reviews aim to identify and summarize available evidence but in a meta-analysis statistical methods are used to combine the results of several studies and produce an overall measure of effect, often reported in a forest plot (see Box 6.1 for an example). Systematic reviews with meta-analyses are usually best for addressing questions regarding the effectiveness of interventions which have been evaluated in RCTs and which have numerically described outcomes (see Box 6.1). On the other hand, in a narrative review, the findings of the individual studies will be synthesized and compared descriptively. Such reviews can be used to describe and synthesize effectiveness studies, particularly evaluations that do not provide numerical results such as the review of housing interventions in Box 6.2 and the review of the cost-effectiveness of African-based HIV/AIDS interventions (Box 6.3). As well as evaluating effectiveness, systematic reviews can be used more widely. For example, they may be used early on in research to provide a comprehensive summary of what is already known and where the gaps in knowledge are, or they may be used to explore and evaluate different analytical approaches to a problem, or to provide the best estimate of the prevalence and population burden of a problem.

Essential characteristics of systematic reviews

The previous section showed how systematic reviews vary in their purpose, structure, and content. However, there are some key characteristics

Box 6.1 Physical activity promotion: a systematic review from the Cochrane Library

To answer the question on how to get individuals to be more active, it was decided to carry out a Cochrane review. Of interest were interventions where advice was directly provided to individuals and where there was some evidence that changes were sustainable. The review was limited to RCTs of adults aged over 16 and not living in an institution. A list of *inclusion and exclusion criteria* was drawn up, for example, requiring a minimum of 6 months' follow-up. Interventions delivered by mass media or targeting adults with disease were excluded.

It took several iterations to develop a *search strategy* that captured the kind of studies that were wanted. Nine *databases* were searched and after removing duplicates there were 35 524 potential titles. To *review the titles and abstracts* each one was considered independently by two people and the full text of the paper was obtained if either reviewer considered it possibly relevant; this lead to 224 full-text papers which were again considered independently by two people. At this point, if there was any disagreement a third person also read the paper and the disagreement was resolved by discussion. Finally, 33 papers were included in the review.

Studies reported many different measures of activity. To *synthesize the evidence* studies were divided into those reporting continuous measures and those reporting dichotomous measures, and separate meta-analyses were carried out.

Table 6.1 shows a forest plot summarizing one of the meta-analyses (forest plots are so called because of the forest of lines that they typically contain). Nineteen trials were combined and the diamond at the bottom shows the overall result combining all the trials and indicates a small increase (0.28 standard mean difference, 95% confidence interval 0.15, 0.41) in physical activity. The conclusion was that 'interventions designed to increase physical activity can lead to moderate short and mid-term increases in physical activity, at least in middle age' (Foster *et al.* 2005).

Table 6.1 Forest plot summarizing one of the meta-analyses discussed in Box 6.1. Reproduced from Foster et al. (2005), with permission.

Review: Interventions for promoting physical activity

Comparison: 1 Pooled effects

Outcome: 1 Studies with continuous data for self-reported physical activity

Study or subgroup	Treatment N	Mean(SD)	Control N	Mean(SD)	Std. Mean Difference IV, Random, 95% CI	Weight	Std. Mean Difference IV, Random, 95% CI
Calfas 2000	160	255.36 (19.57)	155	253.05 (19.35)		6.0%	0.12 [−0.10, 0.34]
Cunningham 1987	111	138.4 (149.5)	105	84.7 (116.3)		5.5%	0.40 [0.13, 0.67]
Elley 2003	451	9.76 (42.26)	427	0.37 (57.03)		6.8%	0.19 [0.06, 0.32]
Goldstein 1999	158	12.58 (72.77)	154	111.03 (68.87)		6.0%	0.02 [−0.20, 0.24]
Green 2002	128	5.37 (1.59)	128	4.98 (1.59)		5.8%	0.24 [0.00, 0.49]
Hillsdon 2002	1095	124 (143.2)	561	113 (229.5)		7.0%	0.06 [−0.04, 0.16]
Inoue 2003	43	4.11 (2.71)	41	3.43 (2.97)		4.0%	0.24 [−0.19, 0.67]
King 1988a	27	11.4 (6)	20	7.5 (6)		2.8%	0.64 [0.05, 1.23]
King 1988b	27	12.4 (6)	21	9.8 (8)		2.9%	0.37 [−0.21, 0.94]
Kriska 1986	114	1514 (1070)	115	1035 (646)		5.6%	0.54 [0.28, 0.80]
Marshall 2003a	227	3.33 (3.37)	235	3.13 (3.39)		6.4%	0.06 [−0.12, 0.24]

Favours control   −1   −0.5   0   0.5   1   Favours treatment

Heterogeneity: Tau^2 = 0.06; Chi^2 = 109.31, df = 18 (P<0.00001); I^2 =84%

Test for overall effect: Z = 4.29 (P = 0.000018)

Table 6.1 (continued) Forest plot summarizing one of the meta-analyses discussed in Box 6.1. Reproduced from Foster *et al.* (2005), with permission.

Review: Interventions for promoting physical activity

Comparison: 1 Pooled effects

Outcome: 1 Studies with continuous data for self-reported physical activity

Study or subgroup	Treatment N	Mean(SD)	Control N	Mean(SD)	Std. Mean Difference IV, Random, 95% CI	Weight	Std. Mean Difference IV, Random, 95% CI
Pinto 2002	112	2 (3.7)	131	1.8 (2.6)		5.7%	0.06 [−0.19, 0.32]
Resnick 2002a	10	31.9 (19.4)	7	18.4 (15.4)		1.3%	0.72 [−0.29, 1.72]
Simons-Morton 2001a	305	33.76 (1.08)	146	33.53 (1.57)		6.2%	0.18 [−0.02, 0.38]
Simons-Morton 2001b	230	32.98 (0.81)	119	32.9 (1.19)		6.0%	0.08 [−0.14, 0.30]
Smith 2000	722	−5.45 (208.55)	373	−22.4 (209)		6.9%	0.08 [−0.04, 0.21]
SSCT 2000	31	43.5 (1.1)	31	42.4 (0.7)		3.1%	1.18 [0.64, 1.72]
Stevens 1998	363	5.95 (2.76)	351	3.64 (2.76)		6.6%	0.84 [0.68, 0.99]
Stewart 2001	81	374 (260)	83	292 (244)		5.1%	0.32 [0.02, 0.63]
Total (95% CI)	**4395**		**3203**			**100.0%**	**0.28 [0.15, 0.41]**

Heterogeneity: Tau^2 = 0.06; Chi^2 = 109.31, df = 18 (P<0.00001); I^2 =84%

Test for overall effect: Z = 4.29 (P = 0.000018)

−1   −0.5   0   0.5   1

Favours control   Favours treatment

Box 6.2 A systematic review of housing improvement interventions

The researchers in this review wanted to know more about whether housing improvements affect the health of people. This is not a research area with any strong tradition of randomized trials and randomization may often be impossible in the context of a political decision on housing investment (see Chapter 4 on randomized trials). Nevertheless, this is an important question with major policy implications.

The researchers carried out an unusually thorough *search*, searching the well-known databases of published studies, hand searching the bibliography of all the documents they found, and requesting information on any unpublished or ongoing studies from subscribers to two newsletters related to housing policy, as well as delegates at an international housing conference. They also contacted academic, local government, and voluntary organizations involved in housing policy.

Because they were not expecting (and did not find) many RCTs, they cast their net widely, including experimental or quasi-experimental studies, but excluding studies that did not adjust for confounding. They established *inclusion and exclusion criteria* to define what they considered to be a housing improvement. For example, they excluded studies of poor air quality but included studies of the installation of heating.

They found 18 completed studies, the earliest dating from 1936, which covered a wide range of different interventions, including, for example, the re-housing of people in medical need, renovating existing houses, and increasing the energy efficiency of houses.

They concluded that the studies were of such poor quality that no conclusions could be drawn. Nevertheless, this review was valuable in describing the available research and identifying serious gaps in knowledge in an area which has enormous resource implication and the potential for significant health benefits (Thomson *et al.* 2001).

Box 6.3 Cost-effectiveness of HIV/AIDS interventions in Africa

In 2002 the options for addressing the HIV/AIDS epidemic in Africa were opening up. Prices for antiretroviral drugs were falling and substantial new funds were available from international donors. Health policy-makers in Africa needed to know how best to balance the conflicting resource demands of strategies for prevention, treatment or care. To address this, an international group of researchers carried out a systematic review of cost-effectiveness studies of HIV/AIDS prevention in Africa.

The authors were careful to collect all available relevant information. They carried out a *search* of several relevant databases, and searched the citation and references of all the relevant papers they found. This is a topic where many reports (for funders of an intervention for example) may have gone unpublished, so they also sought help from experts in the field to identify unpublished reports. The studies they identified were varied, and the authors devised a three-stage process to assess whether to include a study in the systematic review. The first stage applied predetermined *inclusion and exclusion criteria*, such as whether the study included both costs and effectiveness. In the second stage they excluded studies if the treatments were no longer relevant (for example, long-course zidovudine to prevent mother–child transmission). In the third stage they considered whether any relevant and important interventions were missing from the included studies and identified two: the promotion of female condoms and highly active antiretroviral treatment. Although studies of these two topics did not meet their inclusion criteria they included the interventions in the review, using what cost and effectiveness data they could find.

They reported their findings as the cost per disability-adjusted life year (DALY) gained. There was a range of cost-effectiveness. Improving the safety of blood transfusion cost as little as $3 per DALY, and condom distribution to sex workers, combined with treatment of their sexually transmitted diseases, cost as little as $1 per DALY. Single-dose nevirapine to prevent mother–child transmission cost up to $10 per DALY. At the other end of the spectrum, antiretroviral therapy for adults cost $1100 per DALY (Creese *et al.* 2002).

Box 6.4 Key characteristics of a systematic review

♦ Relevant, important, and answerable question

♦ Systematic and reproducible search for literature

♦ Criteria for including studies is stated

♦ Quality appraisal of included studies

♦ Synthesis of findings (narrative or quantitative)

♦ Results of searching and selecting studies reported

that should always be present in a systematic review and these are shown in Box 6.4.

The research question could be about the effectiveness of an intervention (does this intervention work?), or a more exploratory question (what is known about this exposure in this population?). The question should be worth answering, so it must be relevant and important, but it is also very important that the question is *answerable*. This may be obvious, but it can often be challenging to develop a question which is answerable. The PICO mnemonic (Box 6.5) may help in constructing a question.

The next step is to search systematically for the relevant information. The search should be as comprehensive and wide-ranging as possible within the resources available, and should include a search of publication databases, such as Medline, but may also include other strategies such as consulting experts to identify un-published data. The review described in Box 6.2 was looking very widely for interventions that may not have been reported in peer-reviewed journals and therefore used a wide variety of search strategies. By contrast, the meta-analysis described in Box 6.1 included only RCTs, and relied principally on searches of electronic databases of peer-reviewed publications. Whatever search strategy is used, it should be sufficiently described in the report of the systematic review so that it can be reproduced.

After searching is completed there will be many studies which are not relevant to the research question. The next task is to decide which

Box 6.5 Constructing PICO questions

The PICO mnemonic is a useful tool to help construct an answerable question. The question should have four components: *P*opulation, *I*ntervention, *C*omparison, *O*utcome.

Population

Which individuals is this relevant to? The more clearly this is defined the easier it will be to identify relevant studies.

Examples   Children aged 5–12 years and living in Quebec; men who have worked underground in coal mines for at least 12 months consecutively.

Intervention

What is it that is happening to the population? This could be a voluntary or involuntary environmental or individual exposure that can be observed, or it could be an intervention, either initiated for the research or initiated for other reasons.

Examples   Environmental: living close to a busy road, exposure to ambient noise; Individual: diagnosis of hypertension, experiencing intimate partner violence, smoking; Interventional: provision of subsidized-cost cycle helmets, education on how to eat healthily.

Comparison

What is the intervention to be compared to? If we want to know whether something is 'better' we must be clear on with what it is being compared. The comparison may be the opposite of the intervention, but it may be another intervention.

Examples   Living in a rural area (as opposed to near a busy road); having no experience of intimate partner violence; not providing subsidized-cost cycle helmets.

Outcome

Although the ultimate aim might be to 'improve health' or 'increase happiness' these outcomes cannot be described and compared in any meaningful way. The outcome measure should be relevant,

Box 6.5 Constructing PICO questions *(cont)*

reliable, and repeatable but may or may not be an attribute that can have a number attached to it.

Examples   Percentage of school children who have a confirmed diagnosis of asthma; proportion of women reporting their domestic environment feels safe; mean EQ-5D (EuroQol; a validated measure of quality of life) score of the population.

studies to include and to do this inclusion and exclusion criteria are needed. These will reflect the research question and will aim to remove irrelevant studies while ensuring that no relevant studies are excluded. For example, the systematic review of housing interventions in Box 6.2 excluded interventions to improve the indoor environment through furniture or indoor equipment. There are four important reasons why it is essential to have pre-defined inclusion criteria. Inclusion criteria ensure that everyone working on the review will have consistent guidance on which studies to include, that the methods are reproducible, and that those appraising and combining studies do not end up trying to cope with a jumble of relevant and irrelevant material. Finally, clear inclusion criteria mean that people using the review can see clearly what was included and can therefore judge whether the review is relevant to their question. For example, someone wanting to know about the effects of replacing old furniture with fire-resistant furniture would know that the review in Box 6.2 was not relevant.

The studies finally included in the review will vary in quality. Evidence from good-quality studies should carry more weight than evidence from poorer-quality ones and it is important, therefore, to have some indication of the quality of the individual studies. There are many checklists available for quantitative studies (Downs and Black 1998, Moher *et al.* 1999) but there is still considerable debate about the best way of systematically evaluating the quality of qualitative studies (Petticrew and Roberts 2005). Most of these checklists will assign a numerical value to several different aspects of the study and will then summarize those values to provide a single quality score.

However, the concept of allocating one 'quality score' has been criticized because such an overall score may hide more than it reveals. Two papers with identical scores may have completely different weaknesses and strengths. Many systematic reviews now give a table showing how studies compared on each component of a quality score, to enable to reader to make a better-informed judgement.

There are no rules for synthesizing studies in a systematic review. In a meta-analysis there may be an obvious structure to the synthesis, but even then there are many decisions to be made that are a matter of judgement. For example, authors may decide that there are particular characteristics of the included interventions that potentially influence effectiveness and should be explored by stratifying the analysis. Carrying out a narrative synthesis is even more a matter of judgement and will probably involve a lot of thought and discussion amongst the authors. Whatever decisions are made, it is important that the authors are as explicit as possible about the decisions that were made and the rationale behind them.

The methods of systematic reviews should be as transparent as possible, and should show how the literature was searched and how studies were selected. A useful tool for doing this is a so-called QUOROM figure. These figures were originally devised for the reporting of meta-analyses of RCTs (Moher *et al.* 1999)—hence QUOROM, or *Qu*ality *of R*eporting *of M*eta-analyses—but are now used more generally for reporting the results of any systematic review. The exact content of the boxes in the QUOROM figure varies, but the key characteristic is that the QUOROM figure should enable a reader to understand the whole process of the review from the initial literature searches to the final selection of studies to include in the review. Figure 6.1 shows an example of what might be in a QUOROM figure.

Special considerations for systematic reviews of health promotion interventions

Reviews of health promotion interventions should also reflect the underpinning philosophy of health promotion and a group of experts (Jackson *et al.* 2005) have listed additional questions that should be considered in the synthesis of any health promotion review (Box 6.6).

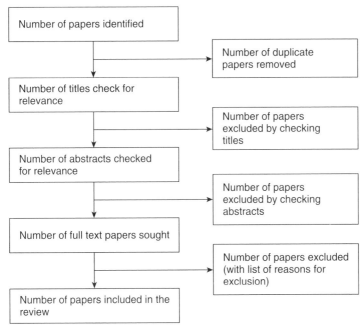

Fig. 6.1 Outline of a QUOROM figure

Box 6.6 Questions for systematic reviews in health promotion

1. What was the theoretical framework that formed the basis of the interventions, if any?

2. Is there evidence on how closely the interventions that were delivered matched the intended interventions?

3. What was the effect of the interventions in populations with differing levels of disadvantage? Is there any evidence about whether the interventions increased or decreased health inequalities?

4. Were the interventions sustainable? Is there evidence of long-term follow-up or evaluation at multiple time points?

5. To what extent did the context in which the intervention took place affect the effectiveness of the intervention?

Adapted from Jackson *et al.* (2005).

Integrating quantitative and qualitative data in a systematic review

Reviews of health promotion interventions will often require an integration of both quantitative and qualitative studies to sufficiently explore both measures and explanations of effectiveness (see Chapter 3). This makes it an even greater challenge to synthesize the results appropriately, but the outcome may be an infinitely richer perspective. Box 6.7 shows an example where the two methodological approaches have been successfully combined in one review.

When two systematic reviews disagree

Sometimes similar systematic reviews will reach contradictory conclusions. This does not necessarily mean that one or the other is wrong and exploring the reasons for the disagreement can be enlightening. Box 6.8 shows an example of how a careful examination of five reviews on preventing falls in older people clarified the reasons for disagreement and also demonstrated how narrowly defined questions provide only limited answers and may need to be complemented by reviews with a broader remit.

Finding systematic reviews related to health promotion

Many systematic reviews of health promotion topics will be found by routine database searches but there are also some useful specialist databases. It is impossible to list them all, but two which are particularly relevant are the Cochrane Library and the EPPI-Centre. The Cochrane Collaboration is a large global network of volunteer researchers who carry out and maintain systematic reviews in all aspects of healthcare. While the emphasis has been primarily on clinical care, there is a specialist Cochrane Collaboration 'field' focused on health promotion, and there are reviews on aspects of behaviour change and disease prevention throughout the Library, including the review in Box 6.1. The Cochrane Library (<http://www3.interscience.wiley.com/cgi-bin/mrwhome/106568753/HOME?CRETRY=1&SRETRY=0>) is available free in many countries or regions around the world due to funding from external sponsors.

Box 6.7 Integrating qualitative and quantitative research in a systematic review

A review of interventions to increase fruit and vegetable consumption in children aimed to examine both quantitative and qualitative evidence (Thomas *et al.* 2004). The aim was to find out what is known about the barriers to, and facilitators of, children aged 4–10 eating fruit and vegetables. The authors carried out searches for both controlled trials and qualitative studies.

They found 33 trials and judged 21 to be of sufficient quality. They carried out a meta-analysis, pooling effect sizes for six outcomes. On average the interventions increased children's fruit and vegetable consumption by half a portion a day. However, there was great variability between the trials with one trial achieving an increase of nearly two portions a day.

They found eight qualitative studies and judged five to be of sufficient quality. The results were synthesized by analysing the authors' findings from the studies using guidelines for thematic analysis. By discussion between three reviewers they identified a number of themes including that children do not see their personal health as their responsibility but that of their parents, and that children prioritize taste over health. Another theme was that children do not regard fruit and vegetables as the same kind of food. The implications of the thematic analysis was, for example, that promotions of fruit and vegetables should not emphasize health but should focus on taste, and that different interventions should be used for the promotion of fruit and vegetables.

The authors of the systematic review then went on to combine the two analyses by checking which of the recommendations from the qualitative review had been followed in the intervention studies. By doing this they identified gaps in the research such as that none of the trials had attempted to promote fruit and vegetables separately. Some recommendations had been followed. For example, eight trials provided information the emphasis of the message and two of the eight had little or no emphasis on health. Those two trials were the only two of the eight to demonstrate a significant effect in increasing vegetable intake.

The authors concluded 'the conclusions of reviews may be substantially altered by the inclusion of qualitative data. . . . This is turn could lead to the development of more appropriate and effective interventions.' (Thomas *et al.* 2004, p. 1012).

Box 6.8 Contradictory systematic reviews

Researchers carried out a study to understand why different reviews of interventions to prevent falls in older people reached different conclusions (Oliver *et al.* 1999). They found five systematic reviews and one 'expert opinion' review.

Different inclusion decisions

One hundred and thirty seven studies were included in at least one of the reviews, but only 33 of those were common to at least two reviews and only two studies were included in all six reviews. The differences were explained by the fact that reviews addressed slightly different questions, used differing inclusion and exclusion criteria, and had different criteria for assessing the quality of included studies (so, for example, some reviews explicitly excluded studies that other reviews included).

Different search strategies

Later reviews built on the references of earlier reviews but invested more resources in searching the literature and found additional trials that the earlier reviews had missed. Although the conclusions of the five systematic reviews differed, all the authors recommended caution in interpreting the results and all concluded that the evidence was limited. Reviews focused on a narrowly defined question only provided limited answers and failed to identify broader research gaps.

Authors' recommendations

- Narrowly defined reviews, often those with clinically defined questions, should be complemented by reviews which take a broader perspective and might include non-randomized studies.
- The methods of carrying out a review should be described clearly.
- Criteria used for assessing methodological quality should be explicit.
- Investment in thorough literature searching is important.

The Evidence for Policy and Practice Information and Co-ordinating Centre (EPPI-Centre) is also a valuable source of health promotion reviews. It was set up in 1993 with the aim of making accessible research findings in the areas of education, health promotion, employment, and social care. Funding comes from a variety of sources including government departments, charities, and other organizations. The EPPI-Centre website (<http://eppi.ioe.ac.uk>) hosts an Evidence Library which provides full reports of reviews conducted or supported by the EPPI-Centre and also Knowledge Pages which bring together key messages from various reviews in a broad topic area, thus providing an overview of the evidence. It provides one of the richest single sources of reviews in health promotion. Whereas Cochrane Reviews tend to be focused on RCTs, and are therefore quite limited in the topics addressed, the EPPI-Centre reviews take a broader approach, in many instances including qualitative research. Boxes 6.7 and 6.8 are examples of work undertaken by the EPPI-Centre.

In conclusion, systematic reviews have an important role to play in assembling and evaluating the evidence of effectiveness in health promotion; a role that is not limited to quantitative analysis of RCTs but offers wider opportunities to understand findings and identify research gaps.

Key points

- Systematic reviews provide reliable, transparent syntheses of evidence.
- The syntheses can involve a meta-analysis or may be a narrative synthesis.
- Systematic reviews can be used to evaluate effectiveness, and also for many other purposes.
- They can include quantitative or qualitative data, or both.
- Health promotion philosophy should guide systematic reviews of health promotion interventions.

References

Creese, A., Floyd, K., Alban, A., and Guinness, L. (2002) Cost-effectiveness of HIV/AIDS interventions in Africa: a systematic review of the evidence. *Lancet* **359**, 1635–42.

Downs, S.H. and Black, N. (1998) The feasibility of creating a checklist for the assessment of the methodological quality both of randomised and non-randomised studies of health care interventions. *Journal of Epidemiology and Community Health* **52**, 377–84.

Foster, C., Hillsdon, M., and Thorogood, M. (2005) Interventions for promoting physical activity. *Cochrane Database of Systematic Reviews* **1**, CD003180.

Jackson, N., Waters, E., and Guidelines For Systematic Reviews In Health Promotion And Public Health Taskforce (2005) Criteria for the systematic review of health promotion and public health interventions. *Health Promotion International* **20**, 367–74.

Moher, D., Cook, D.J., Eastwood, S. *et al.* (1999) Improving the quality of reports of meta-analyses of randomised controlled trials: the QUOROM statement. *Lancet* **354**, 1896–1900.

Oliver, S., Peersman, G., Harden, A., and Oakley, A. (1999) Discrepancies in findings from effectiveness reviews: the case of health promotion for older people in accident and injury prevention. *Health Education Journal* **58**, 66–77.

Petticrew, M. and Roberts, H. (2005) How to appraise the studies: an introduction to assessing study quality. *In Systematic Reviews in the Social Sciences: A Practical Guide*, pp. 125–63. Blackwell Publishing, Malden, MA.

Thomas, J., Harden, A., Oakley, A. *et al.* (2004) Integrating qualitative research with trials in systematic reviews. *British Medical Journal* **328**, 1010–12.

Thomson, H., Petticrew, M., and Morrison, D. (2001) Health effects of housing improvement: systematic review of intervention studies. *British Medical Journal* **323**, 187–90.

Chapter 7

Process evaluation: understanding how and why interventions work

David Ellard and Suzanne Parsons

A process evaluation aims to answer questions about the process of implementing interventions and to place outcome results or the results of trials of complex interventions into context. This helps to support the development of increasingly effective behaviour-change interventions by not only measuring primary outcomes such as changes in health behaviour but also understanding how the intervention has (or has not) brought about change. To understand how and why interventions work we need to evaluate the process of implementing them and for this reason process evaluation is increasingly being embedded into outcome evaluation study designs. This is especially so for randomized controlled trials (RCTs) testing complex interventions (see Chapter 4 for an explanation of RCTs). However, process evaluations are used in many other forms of intervention study, although sometimes called by other names such as monitoring evaluation or process monitoring. Such evaluations are underreported in published literature but potentially provide important insights.

Process evaluations particularly help researchers understand the causal pathways by which complex interventions might work and sometimes to interpret equivocal results. The shift towards greater evidence-based practice means there is a greater need to know why an intervention works or, if it does not, why not. Process evaluation can facilitate this understanding and should be incorporated into the evaluation of health-promoting interventions/programmes.

Process evaluation examines how an intervention is implemented. It does not focus on measuring effectiveness, but on exploring the workability and integration of interventions. Process evaluation has been defined as:

> Evaluation intended to determine the extent to which a particular program is implemented by measuring the activities and quality of a program, as well as whether or not it is reaching its intended audience.
>
> (Cunningham *et al.* 2000, p. 14)

In this chapter we:

- discuss issues relating to formative process evaluation and process evaluation;
- explore the research methods used;
- discuss the integration of process and outcome data.

The scope of process evaluation

Process evaluation assists in the interpretation of results and can also provide information on the feasibility and acceptability of the intervention to both service providers and users. Process evaluation also contributes to the external validity of an intervention. For example, Geraets *et al.* (2006) argued process evaluation is important in studies of clinical effectiveness for the following reasons:

- to know whether the treatment under study was performed according to the protocol;
- to know whether the treatment is feasible in 'normal' practice;
- to identify needs for improvement of the protocol to facilitate implementation.

It can be argued that these same reasons are also relevant to health promotion and behaviour-change interventions (e.g. smoking-cessation services or drug rehabilitation programmes). Is there consistency in how the programme is being delivered? Can it be delivered in the setting proposed? What is working and what is not?

The scope of what constitutes a process evaluation is broad. Process evaluations are an important part of RCTs, but evaluation of the processes of an intervention is also valuable in many other study designs. In Box 7.1 we give two examples of how process evaluation has contributed to understanding the outcome data in study designs other

Box 7.1 Process evaluations of health promotion interventions

Cancer awareness

An educational programme to increase cervical, breast, and skin cancer awareness for women with low incomes was carried out over a 4-year period in six rural counties in the USA (Cunningham *et al.* 2000). The intervention was targeted at health departments as well as individual women and the community as a whole. It included a range of media and print promotion as well as telephone counselling, presentations in the community, and direct education. A large number of process methods were used in this study, including observations, interviews, evaluation forms, focus groups, and meetings. The authors discuss the challenges of monitoring a programme at a distance. They adopted a formative approach to this evaluation (see later in the chapter for a discussion on formative process evaluation).

The process evaluation allowed regular monitoring of programme components and identified areas needing modification (i.e. changes were made as they learned what worked and what did not work). The health department intervention was not successful; however, the process evaluation highlighted some of the problem areas and pinpointed effective intervention components that could lead to desired result of improved cancer screening behaviours.

Smokey Joe

A process evaluation of the Smokey Joe smoking-cessation service in Scotland illustrates the diversity and range of methods that can be used (Ritchie *et al.* 2007). The paper takes an unusual 'narrative' qualitative approach, giving a 'voice' to individual participants (including the smokers and therapists). This approach does not fit easily into the traditional framework for process evaluations, although we argue later that giving a voice to key stakeholders should be considered when designing a process evaluation.

Box 7.1 Process evaluations of health promotion interventions *(cont)*

This evaluation aimed to make clear the assumptions shaping the practice of smoking-cessation groups and assess the smokers' perceptions of the intervention in their attempt to quit smoking. Methods included observation of groups in low-income communities in Scotland, debriefing sessions with facilitators, and interviews with a purposive sample of clients. Results of the observations gave important information about the reach, dose delivered, and the dose received. Intensive analysis of field notes and interviews was carried out and gave a unique insight into the assumptions that shape the practice of smoking-cessation programmes.

Results challenge current guidelines for the length of programmes, suggesting that 6–8 weeks is insufficient and that smokers' intention to change is unstable and requires longer and more flexible support. The paper presents an important message to developers of programmes. The notion that one size fits all is not always valued by participants in the programme.

than RCTs. The methods used and the challenges faced are very similar and in most cases are transferable to process evaluations embedded within RCTs.

There is no simple overall approach to how to carry out a process evaluation. In most cases a mixed-methods approach is most useful where qualitative and quantitative methods are used, including:

- interviews, focus groups, observations, text analysis, and field notes are methods that may be employed to explore the organization of the intervention, the resources, inputs or facilities used, the facilitators and barriers to participation, and the impact of the intervention on the wider health care system (e.g. service use);

- quantitative (statistical) methods are used to explore the 'reach' and 'dose delivered' of the intervention; for example, attendance registers, satisfaction surveys, and surveys of exposure to communications campaigns.

These methods are discussed in more detail in the following section on determining the most appropriate methods.

A sound process evaluation helps with the interpretation of results and in placing these results into context. This in turn helps health professionals and researchers consider how complex interventions interact with existing patterns of service organization, professional practice, and professional–patient interaction (May *et al.* 2007). Oakley *et al.* (2006) have argued that process evaluations have a role in improving the science of many RCTs and have proposed an outline framework for process evaluation in RCTs of complex interventions (see Box 7.2).

Components of a process evaluation

Seven components for a process evaluation have been described by Steckler and Linnan (2002) (see Box 7.3) which show the need to include a wide exploration of the various aspects of implementation.

A recurring message in this book is the importance of planning an evaluation carefully and setting out to answer specific questions using appropriate methods. Steckler and Linnan argue that questions about reach, dose, and fidelity should always be considered. This then raises the question of which other of these key components should be included in the design. These components are very broad and at times may not cover all of the areas that are needed in an evaluation. A prescriptive automated route to monitor processes forgets that

---

Box 7.2 A framework for process evaluation in RCTs

◆ Process evaluation should be integral to the design of RCTs.

◆ Process evaluations should specify prospectively a set of process research questions.

◆ Before the study starts the process evaluators should identify:

  • the processes to be studied;

  • the methods to be used; and

  • procedures for integrating process and outcome data.

Oakley *et al.* (2006, p. 415)

Box 7.3 Key process-evaluation components

Component	Definition
Context	Aspects of the larger social political and economic environment that may influence implementation
Reach	The proportion of the intended target audience that participates in the intervention
Dose delivered	The number/amount of intended units of each intervention or component provided
Dose received	The extent to which participants actively engage/interact with the recommended resources
Fidelity	The extent to which the intervention was delivered as planned
Implementation	A composite score that indicates the extent to which the intervention has been implemented as planned
Recruitment	Procedures used to approach and attract participants

Adapted from Steckler and Linnan (2002).

health promotion programmes and clinical trials are not machines and have a heart made up of the people that participate and the facilitators and researchers who all have a stake in how well a programme is implemented and received. In many cases it may be more important to know what these stakeholders think about the programme and how it has been implemented. Smokey Joe (Box 7.1) illustrates an unusual approach to process evaluation that gives a voice to the main stakeholders. It highlights the important messages that can be learned by engaging with stakeholders and unpacking their perceptions.

Formative process evaluation

Formative process evaluation is principally used during the development (or pilot) stage of an intervention, identifying problems and providing information on changes to improve processes, methods, and procedures and adopts similar methods to general process evaluation. The formative evaluation of the Older Peoples Exercise in Residential Accommodation (OPERA) trial is described in Box 7.4.

Formative evaluation is extremely useful while developing the protocol for an RCT, since most RCTs do not allow for major changes to protocols once the trial has begun, as it leads to inconsistency. Formative or mid-term evaluations during the implementation of other programmes may help to modify implementation and maximize success. For example, such evaluation may identify why a programme is not reaching its intended audience. When evaluating an intervention it can be valuable to feedback data to inform the development of the programme during implementation, to maximize its impact. Action research methodologies involve ongoing feedback that can modify an intervention or programme during its delivery.

Determining the most appropriate methods

Considerations when planning a process evaluation include the resources required. Funding for process evaluators is increasing but is not given high priority, which may limit the scope of process evaluations. However, even with limited resources it is possible to carry out an effective process evaluation that will answer questions about the implementation of your programme or intervention. Limited resources can mean that the process evaluator has a dual role as part of the outcome evaluation team. Not having a dedicated team for process evaluation is a challenge for those working on an RCT as it is important to maintain a distance from the main trial as knowledge of process evaluation findings could bias the trial outcomes.

The scope of a process evaluation often needs a wide variety of evaluation methods. As with all research, the research question(s), processes to be studied, and methods to be used, should be documented at the design stage. Most important is an analysis plan determined at the design stage; including the procedures for integrating the process and outcome data. This is where a backwards evaluation approach (see Chapter 3) can be effective, in deciding what decisions need to be taken on the basis of the process evaluation. Once the goal of the evaluation has been established, the most appropriate methods for collecting the information needed will be clear.

Box 7.4 Formative process evaluation of the OPERA trial

The Older Peoples Exercise in Residential Accommodation (OPERA) RCT is currently testing whether increasing physical activity among elderly people in residential accommodation will be effective in reducing the prevalence of depression (which is usually very high in such homes). The intervention involves changing the culture of the care home as well as providing formal exercise classes. We (the authors of this chapter) are involved in carrying out a process evaluation alongside the trial.

Before the main trial started, a pilot study was carried out in three homes, and was accompanied by a formative process evaluation. We spent time in the pilot homes observing the home routines as well as the activities of the intervention team. We also interviewed staff and residents and members of the intervention team. Although our role was that of a non-participant observer, it was not possible to remain 'non-participant' in such an environment; at the very least, residents expect friendly social interaction. This tension is discussed later on.

The pilot study showed it was possible to recruit participants into the trial and to deliver the intervention. However, the formative process evaluation highlighted a number of issues which shaped the format of the study's and process evaluation's protocols in three main ways.

Methodological issues

- Time taken to recruit and assess participants was greater than anticipated.
- How to measure process outcomes (tools to use, questions to ask): piloting led to refined tools.

Care homes as a setting

- Fitting into the care-home routine can be challenging (time for interviews, residents asleep, meal times, activities): this led to the evaluation team accepting time allocated to each case-study home has to be flexible.

Box 7.4 Formative process evaluation of the OPERA trial *(cont)*
Ethical issues
◆ The consent process was too complex, making it difficult for residents to understand: formative evaluation led to simplifying it.

Participant or non-participant observation

Observation fosters an in-depth, rich understanding of a phenomenon, situation, and/or setting and the behaviour of the participants in that setting. However, there can be a fine dividing line between participant and non-participant observation, as described in Box 7.4. Observation of people in real-life settings makes being a non-participant difficult. For example, do the people being observed completely ignore you or do you completely ignore them if they try to engage with you? Participant and non-participant observation can complement each other. Participant observation 'combines participation in the lives of the people being studied with maintenance of a professional distance that allows adequate observation and recording of data' (Fetterman 1998, pp. 34–5). Using participant and non-participant observation within process evaluation can be useful to illuminate processes which may otherwise be missed, such as the interaction of people, the environment, and the behaviour of participants as a group.

Field notes

Field notes are kept by the observer during or shortly after observation. They are a record of what is observed and may also include comments on the feelings of the observer during the process of observation. Observation tools may also be used to observe specific actions or behaviours and there are some validated observation tools. Whereas field notes are predominantly qualitative in nature observation tools can be either qualitative (e.g. text is written as action is observed) or quantitative (e.g. recording the number of events seen), quantifying what is observed. Often, as with the OPERA study, both qualitative and quantitative observations are used.

Purposive sampling

In-depth interviews and observation are time-consuming and it is rare that resources will permit such work over the whole of a study population. One solution is to select a purposive sample for a more intense case study. This is the solution that we have adopted in the OPERA study described in Box 7.4. Of more than 70 homes in the trial, eight case-study homes will be examined in detail, which will include interviews with residents, staff, family members, and physiotherapists. Observations will also measure the levels of activity within the home and changes over time in the general ethos of the home. These qualitative data will be used to explore the recruitment, fidelity, and overall implementation of the intervention.

Focus groups

Focus groups provide an opportunity to bring together a group of people and elicit opinions on a service or delivery of an intervention. Participants may be provided with a short list of questions to consider before the meeting or topics will be introduced by facilitators to elicit both individual and group opinion which are then discussed.

Quantitative data

Not all process-evaluation questions can be answered using qualitative methods; quantitative methods may be needed to determine the coverage and reach of an intervention and how much people actually received. For example a media campaign may have a national reach but only be received by a smaller proportion. Some people may see the campaign more than others so they get a higher 'dose' of the intervention. These data may be required to answer questions about key components of the process evaluation and how this information is to be collected should be planned in detail at the design stage of the evaluation. The cost of collecting quantitative data depends on the scale of the intervention and the sample size. It is important to have a representative sample for the study population. Taking data from only a sample of sites could restrict the value of the process data. Appropriate data-collection tools should be designed or validated tools used and may include questionnaires, surveys, and study registers (e.g. attendance registers).

Case study: the RIPPLE trial

The RIPPLE trial (see Box 7.5) illustrates the challenges faced when carrying out process evaluation in settings such as schools and highlights the need to establish a good working relationship with the research sites. Protocols may be carefully prepared but it is impossible to consider every eventuality. In the RIPPLE study researchers faced challenges about the acceptability of the research and difficulties in standardizing the control intervention.

The findings from the RIPPLE process evaluation show the richness and depth of information that can be obtained (see Box 7.6). Process information such as this aids in the interpretation of the outcome results and enhances the study. These findings provided important insights into the delivery of the intervention that could not have been collected by the conventional outcome evaluation.

Box 7.5 The RIPPLE trial

The RIPPLE (Randomised Intervention of Pupil-Peer-Led sex Education) study was an RCT of peer-led sex education involving 27 English schools, and included an extensive process evaluation (Strange *et al.* 2006). The aims of the process evaluation were:

- to document how the peer-led intervention was implemented in practice, and to describe the status of sex education in the control schools;

- to compare and contrast the processes involved in the provision of sex-education between the experimental and control schools;

- to collect information from schools and participants about the experience and impact of taking part in the study;

- to gather information about the context of the individual schools and how it may have affected the research;

- to describe the experiences and characteristics of the peer educators.

Box 7.5 The RIPPLE trial *(cont)*

The methods used for the process evaluation included question-naires, focus groups, interviews, observations, and researcher field notes. The process evaluation focused on three groups: school staff, peer educators, and students.

Putting the process evaluation plan into practice was challenging because:

- whereas single-sex focus groups were planned, practical and logistical issues (e.g. fitting into the school timetable) meant that they were not always possible;

- it was difficult to establish what the 'normal' content of sex-education provision was in control schools; delivery and content differed and was not documented;

- it proved difficult to observe the planned 10% of the lessons in intervention schools for practical and logistical reasons; in control schools, some teachers did not inform the process evaluation team when lessons were to take place.

Box 7.6 The results of the RIPPLE process evaluation

There was a lot of variability in the way that peer-led intervention was implemented, including:

- variable amounts of training for the peer educators;

- variable number of sessions (dose) delivered;

- low morale in some peer educators;

- variance in topics covered; for example, the emotional side of relationships were less fully covered than sexual transmitted diseases;

- 10% of target intervention population did not receive any peer-led sex education; school factors were very influential in shaping the ways in which the intervention was implemented and received.

Integrating process and outcome data

Where process and outcome data has been collected independently it is valuable to also analyse the data independently to avoid either analysis influencing the other (Oakley *et al.* 2006). This way of analysing the data allows researchers to generate hypotheses that can be tested later when data from the process and outcome evaluation are integrated. For example, process data from an intervention taking place at a number of geographical locations, can be used to explore the context at each site. Sub-grouping sites based on context may illustrate why an intervention worked better in one type of research site than another. See an example of how process data were analysed separately and then integrated in Box 7.7.

Box 7.7 Integrating process data with outcome data

Process data from the RIPPLE trial were analysed in two stages (Oakley *et al.* 2006, Strange *et al.* 2006). First, analysis was undertaken independently from the outcome data. From this analysis three research questions were generated and tested statistically, integrating process and outcome data.

- What was the relationship between trial outcome and variation in the extent and quality of the implementation of the intervention?
- What processes might mediate the observed relationship between intervention and outcomes?
- Did subgroups of students and schools differ in their responses to intervention?

The team employed several strategies to combine the different types of data, including:

- on-treatment analyses;
- a per protocol analysis where students who actually received peer-led intervention were treated as the intervention group compared with an intention-to-treat analysis (where all students randomized to the intervention are treated as the intervention group);

> **Box 7.7 Integrating process data with outcome data** *(cont)*
>
> ◆ regression analyses and tests for interactions, examining the relation between key dimensions of sex education, subgroups of schools and students most and least likely to benefit from the peer-led programme, and study outcomes.
>
> These strategies provided answers to the three questions.
>
> ◆ More consistent implementation of the programme might have had a greater impact on several knowledge outcomes and reduced the proportion of boys having sex by age 16, but it would not have changed other behavioural outcomes.
>
> ◆ When sex education was participative and skills-based the peer-led intervention was more effective, but when these methods were not used teacher-led education was more effective.
>
> ◆ Peer-led sex education was less effective at engaging students most at risk of poor sexual health; the peer-led approach was better at increasing knowledge in schools serving 'medium-risk' rather than 'low-risk' populations.

Conclusion

There is now an increasing need to carry out process evaluations alongside studies of effectiveness. Effectiveness of a treatment or intervention under study is not only determined by its content but also by its implementation and by the experiences, beliefs, and attitudes of its participants, and their adherence to the treatment or intervention. The design of process evaluation studies, like the design of any research study, is led by the research questions needing to be answered. Process evaluations add value to formative planning, mid-term review, as well as integration into the intervention outcome analysis to provide a greater understanding of the effectiveness of an intervention or programme.

Key points

- Process evaluation examines the implementation of an intervention.
- Process evaluation will help define how or why an intervention has achieved or failed to achieve what was expected.
- Process evaluation research questions should be considered at the design stage.
- Methods used in process evaluations should be designed to answer these predefined research questions.
- Both qualitative and quantitative methods can be used in process evaluation.
- Process data and outcome data should be integrated after the study is complete to provide greater insight into the finding.

References

Cunningham, L.E., Michielutte, R., Dignan, M., Sharp, P., and Boxley, J. (2000) The value of process evaluation in a community-based cancer control program. *Evaluation and Program Planning* **23**(1), 13–25.

Fetterman, D.M. (1998) *Ethnography Step by Step*, 2nd edn. Sage Publications, Thousand Oaks, CA.

Geraets, J.J., Goossens, M.E., de Groot, I.J. *et al.* (2006) Implications of process evaluation for clinical effectiveness and clinical practice in a trial on chronic shoulder complaints. *Patient Education and Counselling* **61**(1), 117–25.

May, C.R., Mair, F.S., Dowrick, C.F., and Finch, T.L. (2007) Process evaluation for complex interventions in primary care: understanding trials using the normalization process model. *BMC Family Practice* **8**, 42.

Oakley, A., Strange, V., Bonell, C., Allen, E., and Stephenson, J. (2006) Process evaluation in randomised controlled trials of complex interventions. *British Medical Journal* **332**, 413–16.

Ritchie, D., Schulz, S., and Bryce, A. (2007) One size fits all? A process evaluation–the turn of the 'story' in smoking cessation. *Public Health* **121**(5), 341–8.

Steckler, A. and Linnan, L. (2002) *Process Evaluation for Public Health Interventions and Research*. Jossey-Bass, San Francisco, CA.

Strange, V., Allen, E., Oakley, A., Stephenson, J., Bonell, C., and Johnson, A. (2006) Integrating process with outcome data in a randomized controlled trial of sex education. *Evaluation* **12**(3), 330–52.

Part III

Evaluation in practice

Chapter 8

Social marketing interventions and evaluation

Steven Chapman

Social marketing was first suggested in the 1950s as a solution to the question 'why can't you sell brotherhood like soap?' (Weibe 1951–2). Marketers were succeeding at increasing use of manufactured products by inventing and bringing to markets brands with new benefits, more variety, and lower prices, which they communicated using packaging and all available communication channels. Marketers had a powerful set of approaches and tools to change behaviour; what if those same approaches and tools were brought to bear on social issues?

Family planning programmes, starting in India and then across many developing countries, were the first settings in which these ideas were tried in the 1960s and 1970s (Harvey 1999). Family planning methods were packaged, branded, distributed in pharmacies and other private-sector outlets, and advertised through multiple communication channels, just like other commercial products. Consumers were not asked to pay the full cost of the product, and most marketing costs were paid by international donors and in some cases local governments as part of efforts to achieve the social objectives of reducing population growth rates and unwanted pregnancies and promoting maternal and child health. Sales of socially marketed family planning products have grown steadily and today deliver a large proportion of the contraception used in the developing world in a cost-effective manner (Harvey 2008).

In the 1980s, social marketing was applied to interventions in the developed world to address risk factors for heart disease, including obesity, high cholesterol, and tobacco use (Lefebvre and Rochlin 1997).

Persuasive communications played a significant role in these interventions, but product distribution was less common. Instead, these interventions emphasized services, such as low-cost medical diagnosis and creating new opportunities for the target audience to get feedback on efforts to change behaviour. These interventions were the first to include evaluation as a core component, leading to the beginning of a social marketing evidence base, and increasingly precise definitions of social marketing's principles and processes. In the 1990s social marketing applications expanded steadily and rapidly to HIV/AIDS and maternal and child health interventions in developing countries, and to a range of health, safety, environmental, and community mobilization interventions in the developed world (Kotler *et al.* 2002, Hastings 2007).

Recently the use of social marketing has grown significantly. In the developing world resources, while difficult to estimate precisely, have probably doubled since 2003, in the range of US$1 billion per year, and are far higher than those available for other health promotion strategies. Nearly every sub-Saharan African, south and south-east Asian country has large social marketing interventions underway, delivering significant portions of condoms, family planning products, mosquito nets, and other products and services. In developed countries, social marketing interventions have become more prominent, particularly in the USA, UK, Canada, and Australia, and are increasingly considered a core tool for influencing exercise, diet, smoking, alcohol consumption, and drug use.

Evidence for the effectiveness of social marketing interventions has also grown rapidly during this period. Evaluations based on cross-sectional surveys routinely report on changes in behaviour and equity and less often on cost-effectiveness and changes in health status. Yet, efforts to review this evidence systematically have had significant problems in determining whether an intervention is, in fact, social marketing. Health promotion experts continue to wrestle with precise definitions for social marketing and for key elements such as a product. Questions have arisen as to whether monetary prices should be charged for products and whether price subsidies undermine commercial offerings and equity. Questions have also arisen about the validity of the behavioural measures used, estimates of health impact, and the strength of the evidence. Evaluating social marketing interventions to influence decision-making is today more challenging than ever before, requiring knowledge and skills from health promotion, social psychology, epidemiology, demography, economics, and health systems policy.

Defining social marketing

Andreasen (1995) defined social marketing as the application of commercial marketing technologies to the analysis, planning, execution, and evaluation of programmes designed to influence the voluntary behaviour of target audiences to improve their personal welfare and that of society. Many other definitions exist, but Andreasen's includes elements common to the others, particularly influencing behaviour voluntarily, as opposed to through regulations, and using commercial marketing technologies. Many health promotion interventions use a single commercial marketing technology such as advertising, and others may use other marketing techniques. Some of these interventions are referred to as social marketing, whereas others are not, posing a definitional problem for evaluations that are interested in determining whether social marketing is effective.

What then makes social marketing distinct from other health promotion interventions? A recent systematic review of the effectiveness of social marketing classified an intervention as social marketing if six benchmarks were met. (Stead *et al.* 2006). The first benchmark requires that the intervention seeks to change behaviour and has specific measurable behavioural objectives. The second states that the intervention must be based on an understanding of consumer experiences, values and needs, using formative evaluation (see Chapter 7 for a discussion of formative evaluation) to identify these, and pre-testing intervention elements prior to using them. The remainder are that the intervention segments its audience, uses a mix of product, price, place, and promotion strategies, offers benefits to the audience in exchange for changing behaviour, and seeks to minimize competing forces to behavioural adoption. The National Social Marketing Centre in the UK (<http://www.nsms.org.uk/public/CSIndex.aspx>) has recently used a modified version of these benchmarks as a framework for case studies about social marketing interventions. This effort and the benchmarking approach generally are important new steps in efforts to distinguish social marketing from health promotion interventions that use advertising or communications alone.

The primary strategy of social marketing is to make practising beneficial behaviours more appealing to populations than competing behaviours that increase risk or vulnerability to disease. Social marketers execute this strategy by choosing what is called a marketing mix of 4Ps: product, price, place, and promotion (see Box 8.1).

The social marketing process consists of a series of steps. The first step is a systematic effort to understand the population's behaviour of interest and the circumstances surrounding it. Next, social marketers iteratively develop the 4Ps based on population preferences first to concepts and then to a more defined social marketing intervention. The social marketing intervention is then conducted, with mechanisms put in place to monitor and evaluate changes in behaviour, perceptions, and potential access. Lastly, one or more of the 4Ps is modified as behaviour, perceptions and potential access change over time.

Commercial marketers have learned that people are motivated, for example, to buy a car when they perceive it to be in their self-interest

---

Box 8.1 The 4Ps of social marketing

- Products are tangible items or services that facilitate the practice of a behaviour; for example, a condom for safer sex.

- Price is seen as the monetary and perceived non-monetary costs associated with both accessing the product or service and adopting the behaviour.

- Place is either physical or the perceived potential access to the product or service or, more broadly, to where the behaviour is performed, such as the home, workplace, school, health centre, store, bar, or community. Social marketing seeks to maximize access and to do so cost-effectively.

- Promotion is persuasive communication, both mass media and interpersonal, regarding the product, service, or behaviour.

and superior to competing offers. Perceived self-interest can range widely, from needing transportation to wanting increased social status. Marketers know that perceived self interests can be shaped by marketing efforts into strong preferences for specific brands and a willingness to spend money and effort and sacrifice other opportunities to buy and own them.

Social marketing uses these same concepts in health promotion interventions. Social marketing interventions aim to compete with those things that people genuinely enjoy or benefit from in the current behaviour, such as the feeling of belonging when smoking with a group of friends who smoke. Social marketers believe that people will voluntarily exchange these perceived benefits for others that are associated with individually or socially beneficial behaviours, but only if the marketer designs and delivers products and services and behaviours that are superior to the benefits being given up. This voluntary exchange marks the measure of success for social marketing and distinguishes it in organizational and ethical terms from commercial marketing (Smith 2001). Box 8.2 gives an example of social marketing in Pakistan.

PERForM: a performance framework for social marketing

The primary issue in social marketing evaluation is the causal association between exposure to the social marketing intervention and changes in the theoretically derived determinants of behaviour, behaviour itself, and health status. Yet, because social marketing also aims to increase access to products and services a social marketing intervention must also be evaluated in terms of health systems performance measures such as cost-effectiveness, equity, coverage, quality, access, and interactions with other determinants of health status. Figure 8.1 depicts PERForM (a Performance Framework for Social Marketing used by Population Services International) which is based on the Behavioural Model of Health Services Use (Andersen 1995) and the purpose of which is to define indicators of social marketing performance.

PERForM has four levels, A–D, with level A consisting of the goal of social marketing for health promotion, namely improved health status or quality of life. Level B consists of the objectives of health promotion

Box 8.2 An example of social marketing in action: the Greenstar social marketing in Pakistan

In 1995, Social Marketing Pakistan and Population Services International, two non- governmental organizations, designed and launched Greenstar and later GoodLife, franchised networks of thousands of doctors, pharmacists, and paramedic health staff working to improve health by increasing the use of contraception and health services.

Greenstar and GoodLife promote their providers as trustworthy, offering high quality, low cost products and services, including advice for men about how to support their wives in choosing contraception. Clinics and pharmacies are heavily branded and advertised through television, radio, and newspapers. Providers receive training, easy access to supplies, and then follow-up support and quality-control visits. In exchange, they agree to comply with the quality standards of the two networks. Providers offer special services to women and men separately, such as the ability to consult a provider of the same sex and offer price-reduced services on special days.

The network expanded greatly the number of places where these products and services are available. Bishai *et al.* (2008) found that the networks provide nearly 30% of the contraception being used in Pakistan, making it the largest private source of supply. Its cost per client is lower than that of government clinics, and the proportion of poor people it serves is higher.

programmes, stated as product or service use on the left and/or the performance of other risk-reducing behaviours that do not involve the use of a product or service on the right. The adoption or maintenance of these behaviours in the presence of a given need is causally antecedent to improving or maintaining health. Level C consists of the determinants (motivations and barriers) of behaviour summarized in terms of opportunity, ability, and motivation and the population characteristics. Level D is the social marketing intervention and other influences or interventions that may have an effect on behaviour.

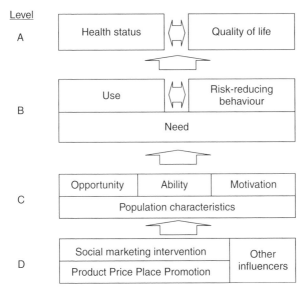

Fig. 8.1 PERForM

Evaluation strategy

At each step of the social marketing process, qualitative and quantitative research strategies are used to evaluate social marketing interventions in terms of PERForM.

Segmentation

Social marketers first *segment* otherwise heterogeneous populations into homogenous groups that are *identifiable* in terms of easily measured variables, *substantial* in size, *accessible* to the intervention, *stable* long enough for the 4Ps to be developed, delivered, and evaluated, *responsive* to the marketing mix, and *actionable* in terms of giving guidance to 4P decision-making (Wedel and Kamakura 1999). The population is divided into two groups *a priori*: those with a health need (including a risk or vulnerability) and those without such need. Those with a need are then subdivided into two further groups: those with a need whose behaviour needs to be changed and those with a need that already perform the behaviour of interest (see Figure 8.2). Those without need are hereafter no longer of interest.

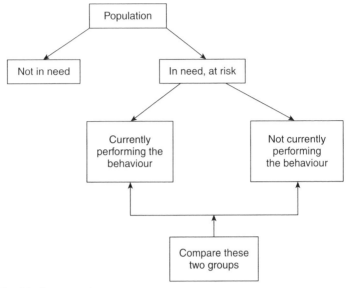

Fig. 8.2 Segmentation strategy

Next, the social marketer makes a *post hoc* comparison of the two remaining groups in terms of level C constructs that are theoretically responsive to the social marketing interventions. The aim is to identify significant differences between the two groups in terms of opportunity, ability, and motivation. Opportunity refers to factors that promote or inhibit the behaviour of interest and include measures of access and availability and quality of care. Ability refers to an individual's perceived skills and proficiency at performing the behaviour. Motivation refers to an individual's desire to perform the behaviour. Motivational constructs include attitudes, norms, and self-efficacy, and their underlying beliefs.

Next, the social marketer determines whether correlations between behaviour, given need, and significant opportunity, ability, and motivation constructs vary by population characteristics (e.g. education, socio-economic status, geographic location). The result is the identification of one or more sets of opportunity, ability, and motivation determinants that, if changed in the group that is currently 'not behaving' would lead to behaviour change.

Environmental/market analysis

The second step of the social marketing process is to conduct an environmental and market analysis relating to the level C opportunity construct. The primary aim is to monitor the availability of products and services that promote or compete with the behaviour of interest; for example, mono-therapies for malaria treatment competing with newer combination therapies.

Strategic, intervention, and marketing planning

The presence or absence of significant associations between level C constructs and level B objectives and the results of the environmental/market analysis guide the decision of whether social marketing is a useful strategy for behaviour change (Rothschild 1999). Intervention objectives are then related to changes in levels A, B, and C, given a planned 'dose' of level D exposures. Marketing plans are developed using qualitative and quantitative strategies used to generate and pre-test level D 4P concepts. Ethnographic research is useful here to generate an archetype of the target audience and to develop a positioning statement that clearly identifies the target audience (see Box 8.3), the behaviour to be changed, the behaviour change benefit, and the competition faced. Monitoring and evaluation are then based on the measures of social marketing performance presented below.

Box 8.3 Examples of positioning statements

In Burma, Zaw Zaw is the name given to an archetypical member of the target audience and Pothinyo is a character who behaves in a manner to which Zaw Zaw aspires. The positioning statement says 'For Zaw Zaw, Pothinyo is his advisor about HIV/STIs and trusted friend who likes to have fun but in a responsible way.'

In Romania, Stefan is the name given to the archetype of the target audience. There, inconsistent condom use and regular switching among condom brands were addressed with a positioning statement that says: 'For Stefan the Switcher, Love Plus is the quality condom that gives him confidence at the best value.'

Measures of social marketing performance

PERForM defines seven primary measures for evaluating social marketing performance.

Effectiveness

Effectiveness is defined as a casual association between level D exposures and changes at level C (opportunity, ability, and motivation), level B (behaviour), and/or level A (health status and or quality of life), given need, and adjusting for other influencers of behaviour. For example, in Zambia, Van Rossem and Meekers (2007) found that men with high exposure to social marketing communication about Maximum condoms were more likely than those with low exposure to the programme to have ever used a condom and to have used a condom at last sexual intercourse.

Cost-effectiveness

Cost-effectiveness is defined as the cost at level D of producing a marginal change at levels B and A. For example, every year Population Services International calculates its cost to donors for each intervention, calculating the cost of averting one disability-adjusted life year (DALY), a summary measure of level A health impact (see Chapter 5 for a discussion of DALYs). Globally, its cost is less than $50 per DALY averted, significantly below benchmarks used by the World Bank to determine whether an intervention is cost-effective.

Substitution and halo effects

A substitution effect is a negative, unintended impact in which one behaviour is increased, but use of an equally beneficial behaviour is decreased. In HIV/AIDS programmes there is a substitution effect known as disinhibition in which potentially a campaign aimed at increasing the use of condoms may be effective, but also results in a decrease in risk-reducing behaviour such as fidelity to one sexual partner. A halo effect is a positive, unintended impact in which efforts to increase one behaviour also results in increases in other, positive behaviours; for example an increase in hand-washing following purchase of point-of-use water treatment. The use of the water treatment is the primary objective, but instructions reminding households to practice hand-washing can also result in the halo effect of an increase in this behaviour.

Equity

Equity in social marketing evaluation is defined as the absence of a difference in the use of a health product or service or the practice of a risk-reducing behaviour, given need, across socio-economic strata. Typically, a target audience is divided up into five groups, or quintiles, by income. If the richest fifth practise the behaviour at the same rate as the poorest fifth, then the behaviour is practised equitably. Socio-economic status can be defined by income, expenditure or asset ownership, or other characteristics such as education, sex, and residence (Andersen 1995).

Coverage

Coverage is the proportion of geographically defined areas in which the product or service promoted by the social marketing intervention is available.

Quality of care

This is the proportion of geographically defined areas in which the product or service is delivered in compliance with minimum standards. An example of a minimum standard might be that condoms are available on every city block where young people go out in the evening.

Equity of access

Equity of access occurs when, among population segments with equal levels of need, risk, or vulnerability, there is equal access to products or services.

Improving the social marketing evidence base

Stead *et al.* (2006) applied Andreasen's six benchmark criteria and found 54 social marketing interventions with evidence of effectiveness in influencing behaviours in developed countries relating to alcohol, tobacco, illicit drugs, and physical activity. Importantly, the label 'social marketing' was not a guide to identifying the 54 interventions as only four were labelled as such. Many other self-styled social marketing interventions did not meet the six criteria.

The findings of Stead *et al.* (2006) create a need to replicate their systematic review and benchmarking on social marketing interventions in the developing world, the evidence base for which has grown significantly in the past 10 years. Most evaluations report on the influence of social marketing interventions on specific behaviours, fewer studies report on the other performance indicators of equity, halo and substitution effects, coverage, quality of care, and equity of access. Whether these interventions meet the six benchmark criteria for social marketing is not known, nor is the extent to which other interventions not labelled social marketing might merit inclusion. It is recommended that all published evaluation studies should include a description of the social marketing intervention in terms of these six benchmark criteria.

Evaluations that form an integral part of social marketing interventions use repeated cross-sectional surveys to measure behaviour prior to and after the intervention. This evaluation strategy has many strengths, including the ability to use baseline information for segmentation analysis and decision-making, and because a control area is not required, the ability to intervene in a broad geographic area. However, there are weaknesses to this approach, which include an inability to randomly assign the intervention to geographic areas or individuals. Randomization would strengthen the evidence and create an opportunity to compare social marketing's performance to that of other interventions (see Chapter 4 for a discussion of randomization). Two recent studies, which are described in Box 8.4, demonstrated the use of randomization on social marketing interventions in the developing world and in doing so produced useful evidence relating to pricing, which remains rare in social marketing evaluation. There is considerable need to replicate this study design across social marketing interventions in the developing world. Further, there is a need to increase the capacity of social marketing researchers and evaluators to use randomization to understand the relationship between changes in the product, place, and promotion Ps, behavioural determinants, and behaviour.

Box 8.4 Using randomization in evaluation of social marketing interventions

Researchers from Harvard Business School examined the how much to charge for health products in the developing world (Ashraf *et al.* 2008). They conducted an experiment in Zambia using door-to-door marketing of a popular home water-purification solution. The price at which the solution was offered was randomly assigned. They found that higher prices screened out those households where the purification solution was used less, creating the opportunity to find an optimum between increasing use and maximizing cost recovery.

Cohen and Dupas (2010) used randomization in a study in Kenya to examine the effect of charging for insecticide-treated mosquito nets. They randomized antenatal clinics to offer nets at no cost or at a low cost (still with a 90% subsidy). They found no screening benefit in charging a positive price, and that reducing prices resulted in higher levels of demand for the nets. They estimated that free distribution of nets could save more lives than cost-sharing programmes.

In instances where commercial-brand market shares decline, social marketing brands may be crowding out sales of commercial brands. Social marketing evaluations could be improved if evaluators were to report routinely on the PERForM indicators outlined in this chapter, along with monitoring the market share of commercial brands over time (Chapman *et al.* 2008). Interventions in the developing world have been criticized for being overly concerned about their own product brands and insufficiently concerned about the growth of the overall market, and about increasing the proportion of target populations using commercially supplied products and services. The Total Market Approach to evaluation encourages the social marketer, based on evidence, to adjust the marketing mix to optimize performance, while avoiding crowding out.

In the developed world, new research and evaluation studies have defined and measured for the first time brand equity, which occurs when individuals who are exposed to different brands form associations with them (Evans and Hastings 2008). Commercial firms such as Nike advertise and sponsor events to increase their brand equity, as measured by consumer perceptions about which athletic shoe is the best quality, or which shoe does the customer buy every time. Brand-equity evaluation is needed in developing-country social marketing interventions, which spend considerable resources developing, promoting, and creating awareness about specific brands. Brand equity can guide decision-making early in an intervention particularly in evaluating initial promotional efforts. Over time, it would be expected to influence behaviour and be a useful component in segmentation and an essential component of outcome evaluations.

After nearly a half century of effort, social marketing interventions face basic evaluation questions relating to distinguishing social marketing from other health promotion interventions, and determining whether social marketing is effective and cost-effective relative to those other interventions. Social marketing evaluation stands to make major steps forward in the coming years if the six benchmark criteria and non-routine evaluation strategies based on randomization are used.

Key points

- Social marketing is the application of commercial marketing technologies to the analysis, planning, execution, and evaluation of programmes designed to influence the voluntary behaviour of target audiences to improve their personal welfare and that of society.

- In the developing world, resources for social marketing interventions have probably doubled since 2003, in the range of US$1 billion per year, and far higher than those available for other health promotion strategies.

- Efforts to review systematically this evidence have come upon significant problems in terms of determining whether an intervention in fact is social marketing. There is significant benefit in applying the six benchmarks to identify social marketing interventions.

> ◆ Social marketing performance indicators include effectiveness, cost-effectiveness, equity, halo and substitution effects, coverage, quality of care, and equity of access.

References

Andersen, R.M. (1995) Revisiting the behavioural model and access to medical care: does it matter? *Journal of Health and Social Behaviour* **36**, 1–10.

Andreasen, A. (1995) *Marketing Social Change: Changing Behavior to Promote Health, Social Development, and the Environment.* Jossey-Bass, San Francisco, CA.

Ashraf, N., Berry, J., and Shapiro, J. (2008) *Can Higher Prices Stimulate Product Use? Evidence From a Field Experiment in Zambia.* Harvard Business School Working Paper 07-034. www.hbs.edu/research/pdf/07-034.pdf.

Bishai, D., Shah, N., Walker, D.G., Brieger, W.R., and Peters, D.H. (2008) Social franchising to improve quality and access in private health care in developing countries. *Harvard Health Policy Review* **9**(1), 184–97.

Chapman, S., Rabary, I., Rharinjatovo, J., Yang, H., and Collumbien, M. (2008) *Social Marketing and a Total Market Approach: Performance Measures.* Working paper 81. Population Services International, Washington DC.

Cohen, J. and Dupas, P. (2010) Free distribution or cost-sharing? Evidence from a randomized malaria prevention experiment. *Quarterly Journal of Economics* (in press).

Evans, W.D. and Hastings, G. (eds) (2008) *Public Health Branding: Applying Marketing for Social Change.* Oxford University Press, Oxford.

Harvey, P. (1999) *Let Every Child Be Wanted: How Social Marketing is Revolutionizing Family Planning Programs in the Developing World.* Auburn House, Westport, CT.

Harvey, P. (2008) Social marketing: no longer a sideshow. *Studies in Family Planning* **39**, 69–72.

Hastings, G. (2007) *Social Marketing: Why Should the Devil Have All the Best Tunes?* Elsevier, Oxford.

Kotler, P., Roberto, N., and Lee, N. (2002) *Social Marketing: Improving the Quality of Life.* Sage Publications, Thousand Oaks, CA.

Lefebvre, R.C. and Rochlin, L. (1997) Social marketing. In K. Glanz, F.M. Lewis, and B.K. Rimer (eds), *Health Behaviour and Health Education: Theory, Research and Practice*, pp. 384–402. Jossey-Bass, San Francisco, CA.

Rothschild, M. (1999) Carrots, sticks, and promises: a conceptual framework for the management of public health and social issue behaviours. *Journal of Marketing* **63**, 24–37.

Smith, W.A. (2001) Ethics and the social marketer: a framework for practitioners. In A.R. Andreasen (ed.), *Ethics in Social Marketing*, pp. 1–16. Georgetown University Press, Washington DC.

Stead, M., Gordon R., Angus, K., and McDermott, L. (2006) A systematic review of social marketing effectiveness. *Health Education* **107**, 126–91.

Van Rossem, R. and Meekers, D. (2007) The reach and impact of social marketing and reproductive health communication campaigns in Zambia. *BMC Public Health* **7**, 352.

Wedel, M. and Kamakura, A. (1999) *Market Segmentation: Conceptual and Methodological Foundations.* Kluwer Academic Publishers, Dordrecht.

Weibe, G.D. (1951–2) Merchandising commodities and citizenship on television. *Public Opinion Quarterly* **15**, 679–91.

Chapter 9

Evaluation of interventions to prevent intimate partner violence

Rachel Jewkes

Intimate partner violence (IPV) is a global problem, causing injury and mortality, as well a range of physical and mental health problems, including HIV infection, post-traumatic stress disorder, depression, substance abuse, and miscarriage (Campbell 2002). Its roots lie in the dominant gender order of societies and changing this requires intervention at all levels: societal, community, family, and individual. Prevention is increasingly seen as an important public health activity, but most research has been on victim responses; that is, secondary prevention. Primary prevention has chiefly focused on individual- and community-level change. Relatively few interventions have been developed and evaluated, which clearly points to the tremendous importance and challenges of stimulating research in this area.

Types of intervention

Among the primary prevention interventions that have been evaluated are school-based interventions on violence (the best known of which is Safe Dates; Foshee *et al.* 2004); interventions that focus on men and boys and building gender equity (Barker *et al.* 2007); mass media activities that seek to raise awareness and change attitudes to violence and risk-factor-reduction activities such as reducing problem drinking or promoting anger management or non-violent conflict resolution. Recently evaluated interventions in developing countries have included a programme for women which combined a small loans scheme (microfinance) with a 10-session group intervention in violence and promotion of community action (Pronyk *et al.* 2006) (see Box 9.1) and a participatory intervention known as Stepping Stones used with men and women (Jewkes *et al.* 2008) (see Box 9.2).

A secondary (and tertiary) prevention intervention that has been widely used and tested is often known as 'screening'. It involves case identification through sensitive questioning, provision of a simple message about the non-acceptability of violence, and referral of cases for further support (Garcia Moreno 2002). Other secondary prevention interventions include legislative measures which criminalize gender-based violence and provide for protection orders and compulsory treatment of offenders; shelters for women; self-help groups; counselling and treatment for men who abuse women; and peer-education approaches which change community norms on the use of violence and gender relations.

Box 9.1 The IMAGE study. Evaluating the impact on violence against women of combining women's access to small loans with training on gender and violence

The IMAGE study (Pronyk *et al.* 2006) evaluated a complex intervention combining small loans given through a microfinance revolving credit (fortnightly repayment and renewed loan) scheme with a participatory learning and action curriculum on gender and violence that was provided to women in loan meetings, which took place every 2 weeks. The intervention had 10 sessions, which were provided over about 6 months. There was then a process of identifying natural leaders from among the women taking loans, and further training them on violence against women and community action solutions, and supporting community activism. This was evaluated in a randomized controlled trial (RCT) in rural Limpopo province of South Africa.

Two years after the start of the intervention, experience of physical or sexual IPV in the past 12 months was reduced by 55% among women in the intervention group.

Box 9.2 Evaluating the prevention of men's use of violence against women through Stepping Stones

Stepping Stones is a participatory HIV-prevention programme that aims to improve sexual health through building stronger, more gender-equitable relationships and through this process seeks to reduce gender-based violence. It was originally developed for use in Uganda in 1995 and has been used in over 40 countries. It uses participatory learning approaches, including critical reflection, role play, and drama, draws the everyday reality of participants' lives into the sessions, and is delivered to single sex groups. The programme runs over about 50 hours, provided over 6–8 weeks (Jewkes *et al.* 2008).

Its impact was evaluated in the rural Eastern Cape in South Africa in an RCT that recruited 2776 men and women aged 15–26 and followed them for 2 years after the intervention. In addition to reducing new genital herpes infections, Stepping Stones significantly improved a number of reported risk behaviours in men, with 38% fewer men reporting perpetration of IPV across 2 years of follow-up ($P = 0.05$) and less transactional sex and problem drinking at 12 months. There was some evidence that a lower proportion of men in Stepping Stones reported raping or attempting rape at 12 months.

These represent a wide range of interventions and each one has its own challenges in evaluation. The nature of many interventions makes the research complex. Determining and measuring appropriate outcomes, and attributing effects, are considerable challenges. Transposing interventions developed and tested in one setting to another is often seen as an efficient way to develop knowledge and a means to circumvent some of these problems. Even if an evaluation of an intervention appears to have strong external validity (see Chapter 4 for an explanation of external validity), the intervention should still be tested in each new setting to establish relevance and effect.

Evaluation design: process and challenges

Although posited as the gold standard, randomized controlled trials (RCTs) should be considered a last step in a pathway, as in drug development (Phase III trials), rather than a first-line methodology. This statement does not undermine their potential to make a valuable contribution to knowledge, particularly attribution of effect, but rather, carefully positions it. RCTs that test the achievement of hard outcomes (e.g. violence reduction) and look for this to be sustained in the long term often have considerable economic and opportunity costs for research teams. Their real place is to test interventions that have been shown through other forms of evaluation to be promising (see Chapter 4). The evaluatory process needs to start well before the RCT is conceived, in the development and initial testing of an intervention.

Research into violence interventions needs to start from the first stage of development or when testing a promising intervention for a new setting. Here formative research is crucial and qualitative methods may be particularly useful. With new interventions, initial planning stages involve developing intervention goals (following appropriate theoretical frameworks of behaviour change), intervention approaches and mapping the content accordingly (see Chapter 3 for a discussion on incremental approaches to evaluation). These require a detailed understanding of the dynamics of violence in the target population.

A second stage involves the initial testing of the intervention with a limited subset of the target population. The focus at this point is not on behaviour or attitude change, but on process evaluation; that is, the more limited goals of testing feasibility of the intervention in the time allocated, coherence, acceptability, and the perceptions of the intervention by the target group. Feasibility and coherence are generally assessed by those delivering the intervention, and much can be learnt about an intervention by asking men or women experiencing it how they perceived it and what impact it had on them. This information can also be used later to shape a quantitative evaluation (see the chapters in Part IV of this book, which discuss involving users in evaluation).

Challenges for intimate partner violence research and interventions

Special challenges may arise in research and interventions addressing IPV. One challenge is the established gender order that position men as socially superior to women, and provides legitimacy for the use of violence to assert dominance and punish women. This is deeply embedded in the social practices of a society and receives legitimization from both men and women. It is very difficult to implement an intervention which seeks to build gender equity in relationships, or to respond sensitively to victims, if the implementers are unconvinced of the appropriateness of this or if they believe, for example, that women are beaten because they deserve it.

Interventions should be tested for efficacy (internal validity) in 'ideal' conditions before they are subject to wider roll out and evaluation in other settings. Part of the process of establishing ideal conditions should include giving special attention to the selection of implementers, including their ideas about gender relations. The programme for training implementers (whether health professionals or intervention facilitators) needs to expound in some detail the context and nature of the problem, and to challenge gender attitudes, as well as exploring and working through personal experiences of violence. This requires time. Some of the notoriously unsuccessful IPV interventions have completely neglected these aspects of the problem, imagining it stripped of its emotive elements and rendered a mere medical risk factor or injury cause. For an example of how these issues may be explored in a training intervention see Box 9.3.

Determining realistic impact and outcomes

Expectations of what impact can be achieved by an intervention should be realistic and commensurate with the nature of the intervention. Interventions that seek to change the general climate of gender relations by challenging norms and attitudes, such as mass-media interventions, can realistically be expected to do this in the exposed population, but to expect a limited-duration, general intervention to impact in a measurable way on behaviour may be unrealistic. Interventions that focus on participants in groups for long periods of

Box 9.3 Design of screening interventions for identifying abused women in health services: developing realistic interventions

A review of screening interventions in clinical settings in North America found that most had lasted 1–3 hours in total. These interventions, however, were expected to bring about a sustained change in behaviour of health professionals who had not previously been introduced to gender and health issues. Not surprisingly they have been shown not to be effective (Garcia Moreno 2002). A more considered approach to addressing the same problem in Latin America and the Caribbean was introduced by the International Planned Parenthood Federation, Western Hemisphere Region (IPPF/WHR). After a careful assessment of services and gaps in staff backgrounds, their intervention included training and sensitizing all staff, improving clinic infrastructure to enable privacy, strengthening policies and staff awareness on confidentiality, adjusting clinic policies and patient flows to allow for screening with written questions about violence, providing specialized in-house support, and strengthening referrals. They also introduced policies to ask about gender attitudes during staff recruitment (Bott *et al.* 2005).

time (such as Stepping Stones; Jewkes *et al.* 2008) can certainly be expected to change behaviour in a measurable way in a well-designed study.

With some IPV interventions, determining what may be a realistic outcome is less straightforward. Listening to the women or men who experience the intervention as well as the people who implement is valuable. Screening interventions usually try to: validate the non-acceptability of violence; enable access to support for abused women; and promote safety planning and trigger other help-seeking practices. If sustained and successful they may change community norms, reduce violence and improve women's health and wellbeing. These outcomes will only be visible in the longer term. Evaluation should initially concentrate on assessing the extent to which the more limited proximal goals are achieved, as it is unlikely that longer-term changes will occur without substantial achievement of short-term goals (see Chapter 3 for a discussion on proximal and distal outcomes).

A first stage, proof of concept, evaluation is very useful. This includes a questionnaire which measures a range of possible intervention impacts. Ideally this stage has two study arms, random allocation is not necessary, and a formal sample-size calculation is not done. The focus is on assessing *what* changes (acknowledging that the design does not lead to any conclusive attribution of impact), *how* much it changes by (necessary for sample-size calculations for a trial), and showing initial promise that can justify further evaluation. Follow-up is short and thus there is a risk of rejecting interventions for not show-ing effect at this stage. Qualitative research undertaken with partici-pants going through the intervention can shed considerable light on the processes of change (see Chapter 7 on process evaluation and Chapter 14 on feedback to participants). Only after successful proof-of-concept evaluation is an intervention well placed to be evaluated with an RCT of appropriate sample size and duration of follow-up.

Measuring experiences of intimate partner violence as victims and perpetrators

Quantitative evaluation of IPV is challenging, but has an important role in rigorous assessment of interventions alongside the use of qual-itative methods. It is important to consider the range of potential abuse. Apart from physical violence, IPV also includes sexual and psy-chological abuse and controlling behaviours. Although IPV is often emphasized, controlling behaviours of intimate partners have been shown to be equally important in influencing certain health risks, notably HIV (Dunkle *et al.* 2004a). Initial work developing measure-ment instruments was done with a view to interviewing women as victims, but more recent research with men on perpetration has begun to show that the same measurement principles pertain.

Developing instruments

Internationally, work to develop best practice in violence research (Ellsberg and Heise 2002) and to create instruments that measure experiences of physical and sexual IPV in a way which is both locally valid and allows for comparison across settings has been undertaken. The World Health Organization has developed an instrument for its multi-country study on women's health and gender-based violence, which has been tested in over a dozen countries (WHO Multi-Country Study Core Team 2000). They recommend that questions on physical and sexual abuse focus on discrete acts of violence rather than using broad and potentially charged, subjectively interpreted words. So, for example, a question should be asked about 'kicking' or 'use of a weapon' rather than a general one about 'physical violence or abuse'.

The effects of an act of physical violence lingers after the injuries have healed and often women describe living in a pervasive atmosphere of fear in between the violent acts. There have been some attempts to develop measures of women's subjective experiences of violence and control in relationships that extend beyond the measurement of violent acts. Two notable examples are the Sexual Relationship Power Scale (Pulerwitz *et al.* 2000) and the WEB Scale (Smith *et al.* 1995). Landenburger (1998) described a cycle of episodes of violence followed by periods of remorse accompanied by affectionate behaviour, but then followed by tension-building phases before violence is repeated. Most researchers agree that these elements are found in many abusive relationships, although the cycle is rather stylized. This poses a challenge for people who want to evaluate the effectiveness of interventions. Positive perceptions of change in a relationship may merely be a product of data capture during the partner's remorseful (honeymoon) phase. Better practice in evaluation of IPV would include measures of the frequency of discrete violent acts and a measure of women's subjective experiences.

Problems of recall

The period over which physically or sexually violent acts are measured is critical. If the period of recall is too long, events are forgotten and so there is greater inaccuracy; if too short it may lead to exaggeration of the frequency because episodes occurring outside the recall period are erroneously included. Frequency of abuse is problematic as an outcome measure because few women experience physical violence on a daily or even weekly basis. For many women it is much less common.

Research in South Africa suggests that approximately a third of women who had ever experienced physical or sexual violence from an intimate partner had only had one episode and that a similar proportion of those experiencing it in the past year have only experienced it once (Dunkle *et al.* 2004b).

Researchers recognize the limitations of reports of violence as an outcome because they are subjective. It is very difficult to validate them, and research has shown that memory of violence is not terribly reliable as it is influenced by the affective state of the relationship. Thus women in abusive relationships who feel their relationship is tolerable and decide to stay may recall violent episodes differently to those who do not (Eisikovits and Winstok 2002). In response to this some have suggested that interviews should be undertaken with couple validation. This is problematic for both ethical and practical reasons. One concern is for women's safety, it could expose women to further abuse from their partners if men perceived that they were losing face due to disclosure of violence in the relationship. Secondly, research with couples shows that recall of violent acts differs between them and is critically related to meaning associated with the act, both at the time it occurred and the time of the interview, with both abusive men and abused women minimizing or 'forgetting' violence at times (Armstrong *et al.* 2001). Thus reports of IPV experiences are inherently imprecise. Taking efforts to minimize bias caused by this is important, for example by using standard assessment methodologies and random allocation between study arms in an RCT. However, the inability to blind participants to which intervention arm they are in may still lead to bias in reporting, especially in studies of interventions that are primarily IPV prevention interventions, rather than interventions to prevent IPV but with other goals such as promotion of safer sex.

Psychological abuse is an important dimension of IPV but is even more difficult to measure. Enumerating all acts of psychological abuse is probably impossible. It is not surprising that there is no substantial body of international opinion on how to define or measure psychological abuse. It is generally agreed that shouting, belittling, verbal abuse, and threats of violence are common manifestations, but in some countries other forms of abuse are also common. These may include taking a partner's earnings, evicting her from the home, stalking her, bringing home or boasting about other girlfriends, undermining self-esteem, failing to contribute to maintenance or the household, dictating what she wears, or trying to control her behaviour and movements. Moreover, measuring discrete acts of psychological abuse may fail to capture the pervasive atmosphere created by such acts.

Some IPV interventions carry a distinct possibility that the intervention may provoke further violence. Although some women find that abuse stops when they have the strength to stand up to their partner, others find that such action escalates abuse. This needs to be taken into consideration in intervention design and the evaluation. Many IPV interventions have been shown to have differing short- and long-term impacts (see Box 9.4).

Attributing change to interventions

Research on IPV can be an intervention in itself. The interview process and accompanying messages about the non-acceptability of violence, as well as the provision of referral information that must be

---

Box 9.4 IPV interventions have greater impact on long-term follow-up

Impact of IPV interventions may accentuate over time and it is critical that evaluations are conducted over long enough follow-up periods. A study evaluating the impact on physical IPV of getting a permanent protection order found no effect at 6 months but a significant reduction at 1 year (Holt *et al.* 2002). The evaluation of Stepping Stones found there was a reduction in men's use of IPV at 12 months that was marginally significant (adjusted odds ratio 0.73; 95% confidence interval 0.50–1.06), but this was significant at a 5% level 24 months post-intervention (adjusted odds ratio 0.62; 0.38–1.01) (Jewkes *et al.* 2008). The evaluation of Safe Dates saw an impact on violence reduction 1 month after the intervention, some effect that was not statistically significant 1 year after the intervention, and then statistically significant findings on violent practices 4 years after the intervention (Foshee *et al.* 2004).

given to meet ethical standards (Ellsberg and Heise 2002), constitutes an intervention. Similarly, research asking men about rape perpetration has been shown to generate self-questioning of their violent behaviour (Sikweyiya *et al.* 2007). This is a particular problem in an evaluation of screening by health care workers, as these interventions often require them to ask just two or three screening questions and yet the assessment questionnaire may include 10 or more, which could significantly influence reflections on abuse experiences in the non-intervention study arm. At the very least, this might reduce the intervention effect size and so sample sizes need to be adjusted accordingly.

Problems of attributing a cause to an observed behaviour change pertain to interventions seeking to reduce IPV. Most women in violent relationships are not able to simply leave or stop the violence or they would probably have done so already. The process of taking action may be started by that initial contact with an intervention, a chance to talk with a doctor or nurse, or seeing a billboard message that women do not need to tolerate such behaviours. The impact of these, if seen at all, should be expected to evolve along a slow, spiralling, and convoluted pathway from there and will include exposure to multiple interventions. Experience of non-governmental organizations that help abused women is that clients often want to test the water when they make their first contact, talk about problems, and get reassurance about themselves and only later try forms of interventions such as leaving. Even then, they often go back to their partner multiple times. Some will try to get family members to intervene or they may get a temporary protection order several times, never going on to making it permanent, or they may engage with other legal and social interventions. If women leave a violent relationship, the process often takes several years. Many women do not ever choose to leave, what they seek is for the violence to stop or lessen and again over time this may happen.

A further problem stems from the fact that most interventions focus on the current relationship and yet it is known that women who enter new relationships after experiencing violence often have serially abusive relationships. Ideally evaluations should have long enough follow-up to capture this but in practice this is rarely made possible due to the limitation of funds and resources needed for such a long follow-up.

In summary, research with IPV interventions must start at a formative stage and then ensure that staff have been appropriately selected
and trained to implement the intervention. Only when this has been
achieved can intervention fidelity be assessed and the participants'
perceptions of the intervention be assessed. Qualitative methods are
most appropriate at this stage and good evaluations will listen carefully to the participants' experiences. This process often takes one or
more years, depending on the nature of the intervention, and may be
iterative with false starts, dead-ends, and so forth. This must be adequately resourced if interventions are to be well developed before they
are tested. When interventions have been shown to be robust they
need to be tested in proof of concept studies to demonstrate promise.
In most cases, it is only after proof-of-concept studies that RCTs
should be contemplated, although the greater rigor and longer
follow-up of an RCT may render visible effects which are otherwise
not seen (see also Craig *et al.* 2008 on developing and evaluating complex interventions).

Evaluations must explore multiple forms of IPV and consider both
subjective experiences as well as objective measures of frequency and
severity. Outcomes are likely to be influenced by exposure to multiple
interventions or to important life events. All this suggests the need for
long-term experimental community-based research in live settings
(see Chapter 10 for more information on this) to enable a better
understanding of the natural history of gender-based violence and the
impact of different interventions to be developed. An ultimate goal
for evaluation would be to demonstrate whether concerted efforts to
intervene can result in improvements in women's mental and physical
health and a reduction in IPV.

Key points

- Interventions must be shown to have been adequately
  developed and their potential understood before a major
  evaluation is attempted.
- Subjects of an intervention should be interviewed to
  understand its impact and potential.

- Both subjective and objective experiences of IPV must be measured.
- Sexual and physical IPV and controlling behaviours should generally be assessed as outcome measures.
- Change often occurs over long time frames, so evaluations need to be appropriately designed.

References

Armstrong, T.G., Heideman, G., Corcoran, K.J. *et al.* (2001) Disagreement about the occurrence of male-to-female intimate partner violence: a qualitative study. *Family & Community Health* **24**, 55–75.

Barker, G., Ricardo, C., and Nascimento, M. (2007) *Engaging Men and Boys to Transform Gender-Based Health Inequities: Is There Evidence of Impact?* World Health Organization and Institute Promundo, Geneva.

Bott, S., Guedes, A., and Guezmes, A. (2005) The health service response to sexual violence: lessons from IPPF/WHR member associations in Latin America. In Jejeebhoy, S., Shah, I., and Thapa, S., eds, *Sex Without Consent: Young People in Developing Countries*, pp. 251–68. Zed Press, London.

Campbell, J.C. (2002) Health consequences of intimate partner violence. *Lancet* **359**, 1331–6.

Craig, P., Dieppe, P., Macintyre, S., Michie, S., Nazareth, I., and Petticrew, M. (2008) Developing and evaluating complex interventions: the new Medical Research Council guidance. Medical Research Council Guidance. *British Medical Journal* **337**, a1655.

Dunkle, K.L., Jewkes, R.K., Brown, H.C., Gray, G.E., McIntryre, J.A. and Harlow, S.D. (2004a) Gender-based violence, relationship power and risk of prevalent HIV infection among women attending antenatal clinics in Soweto, South Africa. *Lancet* **363**, 1415–21.

Dunkle, K.L., Jewkes, R.K., Brown, H.C. *et al.* (2004b) Prevalence and patterns of gender-based violence and revictimization among women attending antenatal clinics in Soweto, South Africa. *American Journal of Epidemiology* **160**, 230–9.

Eisikovits, Z. and Winstok, Z. (2002) Reconstructing intimate violence: the structure and content of recollections of violent events. *Qualitative Health Research* **12**, 685–99.

Ellsberg, M. and Heise, L. (2002) Bearing witness: ethics of domestic violence research. *Lancet* **359**, 1599–1604.

Foshee, V.A., Bauman, K.E., Ennett, S.T., Linder, G.F., Benefield, T., and Suchindran, C. (2004) Assessing the long term effects of the Safe Dates program and a booster in preventing and reducing adolescent dating violence victimisation and perpetration. *American Journal of Public Health* **94**, 619–24.

Garcia Moreno, C. (2002) Dilemmas and opportunities for an appropriate health-service response to violence against women. *Lancet* **359**, 1509–14.

Holt, V.L., Kernic, M.A., Lumley, T., Wolf, M.E., and Rivara, P. (2002) Civil protection orders and risk of subsequent police-reported violence. *Journal of the American Medical Association* **288**, 585–94.

Jewkes, R., Nduna, M., Levin, J. *et al.* (2008) Impact of Stepping Stones on HIV, HSV-2 and sexual behaviour in rural South Africa: cluster randomised controlled trial. *British Medical Journal* **337**, a506.

Landenburger, K.M. (1998) The dynamics of leaving and recovering from an abusive relationship. *Journal of Obstetric, Gynaecologic and Neonatal Nursing* **27**, 700–6.

Pronyk, P., Hargreaves, J.R., Kim, J.C. *et al.* (2006) Effect of a structural intervention for the prevention of intimate partner violence and HIV in rural South Africa: a cluster randomised trial. *Lancet* **368**, 1973–83.

Pulerwitz, J., Gortmaker, S., and De Jong W. (2000) Measuring sexual relationship power in HIV/STD research. *Sex Roles* **42**, 637–60.

Sikweyiya, Y., Jewkes, R., and Morrell, R. (2007) Talking about rape: men's responses to questions about rape in a research environment in South Africa. *Agenda* **74**, 48–57.

Smith, P.H., Earp, J.A., and DeVellis, R. (1995) Measuring battering: Development of the Women's Experience with Battering (WEB) scale. *Women's Health: Research on Gender, Behavior, and Policy* **1**(4), 273–88.

WHO Multi-Country Study Core Team (2000) *WHO Multi-Country Study On Women's Health And Life Events Questionnaire Version 9.9.* World Health Organization, Geneva.

Chapter 10

Evaluating environmental interventions through natural experiments

Melvyn Hillsdon

Natural experiments occur when policy or the forces of nature conspire to produce environments where variations in exposure to health-promoting or health-damaging environments are 'naturally' allocated. This might include changes to housing provision, recreational facilities, supermarkets, or transport infrastructure (Angrist and Krueger 2001). They are important as they provide an opportunity to evaluate the effects of the wider determinants of health in real-world settings where randomized controlled trials (RCTs) are not feasible. This chapter explores the relationship between the built environment and health behaviours. In particular, it focuses on the challenges and opportunities for evaluating interventions that have manipulated some aspect of the environment either directly or indirectly for health gain.

Background

In the mid-nineteenth century urban planners and public health professionals worked together to produce changes to the built environment that led to dramatic public health improvements. The focus of the first of the Public Health Acts in 1848 was on environmental conditions such as drainage, removal of refuse from habitations and streets, and improvements to the water supply. Since then the collaboration between public health and the built environment has diminished as interest in the effect of the built environment on health decreased in favour of a greater focus on individual behaviours (see Chapter 2 for more detailed discussion on these historical developments). However, it is increasingly recognized that many of today's diseases and their behavioural determinants are influenced by the built environment. Once again public health professionals are re-establishing their relationship with urban planners to develop public health solutions. At the first global conference on health in Ottawa in 1986 (World Health Organization 1986) key action areas for addressing the determinants of health were identified and included the need to 'create supportive environments'. The Ottawa Charter for health promotion stated that 'the protection of the natural and built environments and the conservation of natural resources must be addressed in any health promotion strategy.' At the fifth global conference on health promotion in Bangkok in 2005 (World Health Organization 2005) a new charter for health promotion reiterated the importance of the environment, suggesting that global environmental change and urbanization are two of the critical determinants of health.

The built environment has been defined as 'all building, spaces and products that are created or modified by people' (Health Canada, Division of Childhood and Adolescence 2002). In practice the focus has been on housing, transport, and neighbourhood characteristics, as shown in Figure 10.1, which illustrates the link between the built environment and health and wellbeing.

Health promotion programmes can modify the determinants of health, which include individual behaviours, heath service use, and environmental, social, and economic conditions. For most of the twentieth century health promotion focused on individual behaviours. In part this was due to the dominant theories of behaviour change which emphasized psychosocial determinants. In the 1990s there was an increase in the use of socio-ecological models that emphasized the interaction between people and place (Stokols 1992). Since then there has been a rapid increase in the number of research studies investigating the association between aspects of the built environment and health. For example, a great deal of research has been conducted on food environments and physical activity environments with the aim of better understanding the wider determinants of obesity (Butland *et al.* 2007).

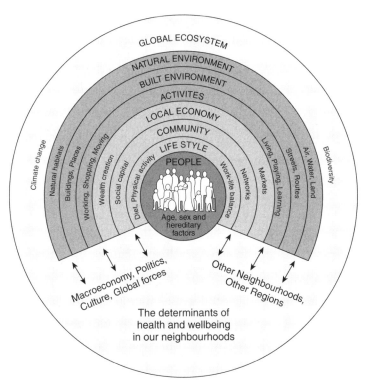

Fig. 10.1 Built environment and health

Reproduced from Barton, H. and Grant, M. (2006) A health map for the local human habitat. *Journal of the Royal Society for the Promotion of Health* **126**, 252–3, copyright © 2006 by Royal Society for Public Health. Reprinted by Permission of SAGE.

Methods of evaluating environmental interventions

Many of the studies evaluating the relationship between the built environment and health have been cross-sectional and have provided evidence of a correlation between a range of measures of the built environment and health. But correlations do not necessarily mean causation. One of the main limitations of correlation studies of the environment and health is the possibility that the correlations can be explained by selection bias. Does a neighbourhood conducive to walking cause more walking or do people with a desire to walk move to a neighbourhood conducive to walking? Much of the existing evidence for a relationship between the environment and health could simply be due to reverse causality. That is, healthy people tend to migrate to more health-promoting neighbourhoods and people who suffer poor health migrate downwards to less-health-promoting neighbourhoods (Cummins *et al.* 2007). In order to better understand the direction of the relationship between the built environment and health behaviours we require more longitudinal studies as well as studies of environmental interventions (Bauman 2005).

The most robust evidence about causal effects comes from RCTs (see Chapter 4 for a discussion of the hierarchy of evidence). However, randomizing people to certain environments or randomizing environmental interventions to specific places, although not impossible, is rare (Sallis *et al.* 2009). Most environmental interventions are not instituted by researchers and the reason for the intervention is rarely health gain. Any effects on health are unintended. 'Natural experiments' occurring in everyday environments, such as the opening of a new supermarket, the building of a new road, or the introduction of a congestion charge, mean that variations in exposure are naturally allocated. Such natural experiments offer opportunities to evaluate the effects of environmental interventions that would otherwise be too expensive for health-funding agencies to consider (Petticrew *et al.* 2005).

There are currently few evaluations of the effects of natural experiments on health behaviours and those that there are have numerous methodological limitations. A systematic review (see Chapter 6) of environmental interventions found serious weaknesses in the methods of the majority of studies (see Box 10.1).

Both non-experimental and quasi-experimental study designs have been used to evaluate the effects of natural experiments. They include less robust designs such as post-intervention-only measures and uncontrolled before-and-after studies as well as more robust designs such as controlled before-and-after studies.

Post-intervention-only measure

This is the weakest of study designs and is only really appropriate in pilot studies where an assessment of the effectiveness of the intervention is

Box 10.1 Systematic review of environmental interventions to promote physical activity

In 2008 the English National Institute for Health and Clinical Excellence (NICE) identified 54 studies that included a measure of change in the environment as part of the intervention and physical activity as an outcome. Fewer than 20% of the studies included a comparison/control group and 35 of the 54 studies only had a post-intervention measure of physical activity. The average length of follow-up was 8 weeks and very few studies collected data on potential confounding factors. Thus the results were poor (NICE 2008).

not required. No causal inferences can be made and findings are primarily restricted to process evaluation, including participants' and providers' views of the intervention. An example of such a study is the study of walking trails in the USA (Box 10.2).

The implicit hypothesis of this study was that access to a trail would encourage use of the trail and trail use would lead to increased walking. The study was cross-sectional in design as the measures for each of these three factors were assessed at the same time. This prevents us from making any inference about the direction of the observed relationships. The possibility that current walkers simply transferred their existing walking routes to incorporate the new trails cannot be ruled out. The sample was selected using a random telephone-dialling procedure and had a reasonably high response rate (73%) which would minimize potential response bias compared to a non-random sampling procedure. The measurement of both the exposure to the intervention and the outcome (walking) relied on self report and both were collected after the intervention had occurred. Attributing the cause of any increase in walking to trail use relied on the participants saying so. Distances to trails and the time since the trail was built varied considerably and both factors are likely to have affected reports of trail use. These factors were not taken into account in the analysis. Further, trail use may have been a consequence of an earlier decision to change physical activity rather than the factor that led to a decision

Box 10.2 Walking trails in the USA

Researchers in the USA evaluated the use of new walking trails provided in a rural community (Brownson *et al.* 2000). At the time of the survey the trails had been in existence for between 6 months and 5 years, so it was not possible to make any measurements prior to the intervention. In the region where the study was undertaken there were 21 walking trails, mainly located in residential parks. They varied in length between 0.13 and 2.38 miles. A random sample of 1269 residents, selected from 17 communities (eight with walking trails in the local area, nine without), were surveyed by telephone interview. Seventy three per cent of eligible residents took part in the survey, which enquired about recent physical activity, including walking, perceived access to trails, use of walking trails, and reported change in physical activity due to trail use. Reported walking-trail use was higher in women than men, higher in higher socio-economic groups, lower in older ages, and higher in respondents who said they were already regular walkers.

Of the respondents who said they used walking trails, 55% also reported an increase in their walking since using the trail. Women who had used walking trails were twice as likely to report an increase in walking as men and respondents who reported using longer trails (half a mile or more compared with a quarter of a mile or less) were more likely to report an increase in walking. Despite reporting more frequent trail use, better-educated respondents were less likely to report an increase in walking since using trails compared to less-educated trail users. Within trail users, current walking frequency and distance to the trails was not related to self reports of increased walking. This may have been partly due to the fact that 43% of respondents were at least 15 miles from the nearest trail.

to change. The fact that some people reported an increase in walking since using trails may simply have been a coincidence rather than evidence of cause and effect.

Uncontrolled before-and-after study (prospective cohort)

In an uncontrolled before-and-after study a single population is measured/observed before the start of the intervention and again at a predetermined time afterwards. The lack of a control or comparison population means that any changes that are observed could be due to secular trends in the population or factors other than the intervention, preventing conclusions about the cause of any observed changes. The traffic-calming study described in Box 10.3 provided some evidence that the introduction of a traffic-calming scheme led to positive changes in health behaviour and one measure of health status. However, selection and response bias may have affected the results. Responders to the initial survey were not representative of the age and sex distribution of the local population and may have been healthier than non-responders. Responders to the follow-up survey may have been restricted to people more likely to have changed. Nevertheless, there was also a positive change in the pedestrian counts that were objectively recorded. If the non-responders had not changed their behaviour and were less healthy then the observed results are likely to have been an exaggeration of the true effect of the intervention. The absence of a control sample means that we cannot exclude the possibility that temporal social and environmental changes explain the changes. It is also possible that the traffic-calming measures on the one road simply displaced some traffic to other local roads and that may have had detrimental health effects. These potential unintended negative effects may balance out any positive changes in the intervention area.

Controlled before-and-after study (quasi-experiment)

In this design there are intervention and control populations that are both observed prior to the intervention and for a predetermined period after the start of the intervention. In environmental interventions, the

Box 10.3 Traffic calming and health status

In a small deprived neighbourhood in Glasgow, Scotland, measures to slow traffic and assist road crossing were built on the main road that bisected a housing estate. A random sample of 750 households was selected from 2587 potential households and were sent a baseline questionnaire by mail prior to the start of the building work. In addition, at three locations on the road, pedestrian counts were recorded before and after the intervention at the same times of the day. The response rate for the baseline questionnaire was 39.1%. Follow-up questionnaires were sent to respondents to the baseline questionnaire who agreed to this. The response rate to the follow-up questionnaire was 32.1%. In both surveys, respondents were older than the local population from which they were drawn and women were overrepresented. The questionnaires included a self-report measure of physical activity as well as a measure of reported health (Short Form-36). In the follow-up questionnaire respondents were asked whether they had done more of a range of behaviours as a result of the traffic-calming scheme. Apart from reported changes to cycling in the area, all other reported changes were significant (Figure 10.2). Pedestrian counts increased between

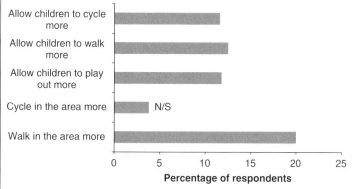

Fig. 10.2 Proportion of respondents who answered positively to the question: have you done any of the following more as a result of the introduction of the traffic-calming scheme?
N/S, not significant. Morrison *et al.* (2004).

Box 10.3 Traffic calming and health status (cont)

the baseline and follow-up measures for all locations and ages apart for some pensioners on one section of the road.

A significant increase in the physical component score of the Short Form-36 but not in the mental component score was observed between the two surveys.

intervention is not under the control of the researcher and therefore the populations are not randomly assigned. This allows for the possibility that any changes observed and any differences in the outcome between the two populations at follow-up may be due to differences in the two populations other than exposure to the intervention.

In the evaluation of the effect of a new supermarket described in Box 10.4 the low response rate to the baseline survey means that there may have been some selection bias, although respondents had a similar age and sex distribution to the local population. Respondents had a higher than would be expected average fruit and vegetable consumption based on other population surveys. Assuming the self reports were not biased, it is possible that the intervention might have had a larger affect if people in the study sample had lower baseline levels of consumption of fruit and vegetables with greater scope for improvement. The positive changes observed in combined fruit and vegetable consumption in both the intervention and comparison areas highlight the importance of the comparison area. The absence of a comparison area may have led to the conclusion that the arrival of the new supermarket had increased fruit and vegetable consumption.

Challenges facing natural experiments

Natural experiments provide an opportunity to evaluate interventions when randomization of populations or environments is not feasible. Natural experiments such as environmental interventions can make an important contribution to the public health evidence base (Wanless 2004) but, as we have seen above, evaluating them is not without problems. The problems fall under four main headings, as follows.

Box 10.4 Access to fruit and vegetables and changes in consumption

A study in Glasgow, Scotland, assessed whether the opening of a new supermarket changed fruit and vegetable consumption in the local population (Cummins *et al.* 2005). A prospective, controlled before-and-after study was conducted in two areas: an intervention area and a control/comparison area. The study areas were approximately 5 km apart to reduce contamination so that the residents of the comparison area were not affected by the opening of the supermarket. A postal survey was sent to a random sample of 3975 households at baseline (approximately a month before the supermarket opened) and 12 months later a repeat questionnaire was sent to households that responded. The sampling frame was based on household postcodes encompassing the main shopping provision in each area and represented more deprived households. The questionnaire included self-reported fruit and vegetable consumption and a self-reported measure of health (the GHQ-12). The response rate was 15.2% for the baseline questionnaire and 68.4% for the follow-up questionnaire. After controlling for differences in baseline consumption and other potential confounding factors, there was no difference in the increases in fruit and vegetable consumption or psychological health between the two areas.

Defining the exposed population

It is difficult to define the affected population in interventions that involve a change to the built environment. As in the traffic-calming example (Box 10.3) environmental interventions can have intended and unintended effects, making selection of the affected population problematic. Should it include just the road and adjoining roads where the intervention is taking place? If traffic is displaced elsewhere, should a wider community be included? What about commuters travelling by car or cycle, or pedestrians who live further away but use the road on their way to work? If there are commercial, educational, or employment premises in the road, should the people who work there and their customers, who may not live locally, be included? Respondents' views on the success of the intervention may be influenced by the population chosen for study and therefore considerable bias could be introduced. Further population influences may include the length of time people have lived in the area and their view of the area's historical context.

The intervention being assessed

In advance of major environmental interventions, such as the building of a new supermarket, it is common for other environmental changes to occur. Access to the supermarket may involve new roads or changes to the existing road network, and public transport routes may change. Natural 'short cuts' that pedestrians frequently use may disappear. In anticipation of the new supermarket, businesses may start to change what they offer or business premises may change hands, affecting the flow of people in and out of an area. In very large developments (such as the preparations for the 2012 Olympics in London), the length of building time may be sufficient for selective migration to take place. For example, the new development may lead to changes in the value of homes and therefore the make-up of the local population. All of these possibilities make it challenging to define exactly what the intervention population are 'exposed' to. It follows from these issues that the timing of when to make the baseline measures is a further challenge. The start date may be delayed, or, if anticipatory changes that are likely to affect the population take place before the intended intervention, determining a start date can be an arbitrary process. In turn, this has implications for applying for money for evaluation since funders' processes do not normally allow for variable start dates.

The selection of a sample population

The selective migration described above has implications for the study design. In the example in Box 10.4, the same people were measured before the intervention and followed and measured again after the intervention. If the duration of the intervention is long or the start date has a long run in, it is possible that many of the people measured at baseline will have moved away. If this occurs relatively soon after the intervention has started is it reasonable to say they have been exposed to the intervention? Indeed, how long does somebody need to be exposed to the intervention before it is likely to have an impact on behaviour or health? The health benefits of reduced exposure to traffic emissions may take years. If it is predicted that population turnover in the intervention area is going to be high then it may be more advantageous to use a repeated cross-sectional design. A repeated cross-sectional study would allow data to be gathered on people who have migrated into the area as well as those who have been there for the duration of the study.

As evidence in the supermarket study (Box 10.4) showed, there are obvious benefits from including control/comparison populations when evaluating environmental interventions. In that study, the researchers tried to identify a matched population that was sufficiently removed from the intervention area so as to avoid contamination. This can be problematic, especially when the intervention is specific to the intervention area (for example the London traffic congestion charge). Ideally, to maximize the study's internal validity the only difference between the intervention and control communities should be the intervention (see Chapter 4 for a discussion of internal validity). In practice, with environmental interventions this is highly unlikely.

The choice of outcome measures

Environmental interventions are usually not undertaken to benefit health or change health behaviour. The primary aim of opening supermarkets, calming traffic, and even building cycling lanes is not usually health gain. Also, environmental interventions typically have unintended as well as intended effects on health. Therefore, identifying suitable outcome measures requires care. Evidence from correlation studies suggest that the effect of an environmental exposure may be specific to certain behaviours (Giles-Corti et al. 2005). For example, 'walkability' of a neighbourhood appears to be associated with walking for transport but not walking for leisure. A general measure of walking would likely lead to an underestimate of the true effect of the environment. There is a lack of evidence-based theoretical models linking environmental exposures to behavioural outcomes and this lack may prevent the development of more sophisticated studies testing explicit hypotheses about the relationship between specific environmental exposures and types of health behaviour (Ball *et al.* 2006).

In conclusion, although not without their problems, natural experiments provide a unique opportunity to add to the public health evidence base when RCTs are not feasible, appropriate, or practicable. Although they have weak internal validity, natural experiments take place in the real world and are therefore not only of policy interest but have a strong external validity. They can help lead to better understanding of the wider determinants of health and health inequalities; and offer greater opportunity for replication.

Key points

+ The determinants of health behaviour and health occur at multiple levels and include the built environment (e.g. the transport system), access to water or healthy foods, opportunities for recreation, and access to health services.

+ Much of the evidence for an association between the built environment and health comes from cross-sectional studies that prevent any inferences about causality.

+ Natural experiments in the built environment provide an opportunity to evaluate the effectiveness of interventions when complex RCTs are not feasible.

+ Natural experiments are often undertaken for non-health reasons but can have intended and unintended effects on health.

+ Results from natural experiments can make an important contribution to the public health/health promotion evidence base; however, they suffer from a range of biases and their evaluation results require careful handling.

References

Angrist, J.D. and Krueger, A.B. (2001) Instrumental variables and the search for identification: from supply and demand to natural experiments. *Journal of Economic Perspectives* **15**, 69–85.

Ball, K., Timperio, A.F., and Crawford, D. (2006) Understanding environmental influences on nutrition and physical activity behaviours: where should we look and what should we count? *International Journal of Behavioural Nutrition and Physical Activity* **3**, 33.

Barton, H. and Grant, M. (2006) A health map for the local human habitat. *Journal of the Royal Society for the Promotion of Health* **126**, 252–3.

Bauman, A. (2005) The physical environment and physical activity: moving from ecological associations to intervention evidence. *Journal of Epidemiology and Community Health* **59**, 535–36.

Brownson, R.C., Housemann, R.A., Brown, D.R., Jackson-Thomson, J., King, A.C., Malone, B.R., and Sallis, J.F. (2000) Promoting physical activity in rural communities: walking trail access, use and effects. *American Journal of Preventive Medicine* **18**, 235–41.

Butland, B., Kopelman, P., McPherson, K., Thomas, S., Mardell, J., and Parry, V. (2007) *Foresight. Tackling Obesities: Future Choices - Project Report*, 2nd edn. Government Office for Science, London.

Cummins, S., Petticrew, M., Higgins, C., Findlay, A., and Sparks, L. (2005) Large scale food retailing as an intervention for diet and health: quasi-experimental evaluation of a natural experiment. *Journal of Epidemiology and Community Health* **59**, 1035–40.

Cummins, S., Curtis, S., Diez-Roux, A.V., and Macintyre, S. (2007) Understanding and representing place in health research: a relational approach. *Social Science & Medicine* **65**, 1825–38.

Giles-Corti, B., Timperio, A., Bull, F., and Pikora, T. (2005) Understanding physical activity environmental correlates: increased specificity for ecological models. *Exercise & Sport Science Reviews* **33**, 175–81.

Health Canada, Division of Childhood and Adolescence (2002) *Natural and Built Environments*. www.hc-sc.gc.ca/dca-dea/publications/healthy_dev_partb_5_e.html. Health Canada, Ottawa.

Morrison, D.S., Thomson, H., and Petticrew, M. (2004) Evaluation of the health effects of a neighbourhood traffic calming scheme. *Journal of Epidemiology and Community Health* **58**, 837–40.

NICE (2008) *Promoting and Creating Built or Natural Environments that Encourage and Support Physical Activity*. National Institute for Health and Clinical Excellence, London.

Petticrew, M., Cummins, S., Ferrell, C. et al. (2005) Natural experiments: an underused tool for public health? *Public Health* **119**, 751–7.

Sallis, J.F., Story, M., and Lou, D. (2009) Study designs and analytic strategies for environmental and policy research on obesity, physical activity and diet: recommendations from a panel of experts. *American Journal of Preventive Medicine* **36**(2S), S72–7.

Stokols, D. (1992) Establishing and maintaining healthy environments. Toward a social ecology of health promotion. *American Psychology* **47**, 6–22.

Wanless, D. (2004) *Securing Good Health for the Whole Population: Final Report.* HM Treasury, London.

World Health Organization (1986) *Ottawa Charter for Health Promotion.* www.who.int/hpr/NPH/docs/ottawa_charter_hp.pdf. World Health Organization, Geneva.

World Health Organization (2005) *The Bangkok Charter for Health Promotion in a Globalized World.* www.who.int/healthpromotion/conferences/6gchp/hpr_050829_%20BCHP.pdf. World Health Organization, Geneva.

Chapter 11

E-health promotion

John Powell

E-health is a term that encompasses the use of new information and communication technologies for improving health and health care. Sometimes the scope of e-health is restricted to web-based tools, but with the increasing convergence of networked technologies across multiple platforms, such as mobile telephony or interactive digital television, a broader definition is more helpful to include initiatives which may perhaps use mobile or pervasive technology. (Pervasive technology is also referred to as ubiquitous computing. It describes the integration of computing power into everyday objects and activities. For example, bathroom scales can be used by a health care provider to remotely monitor a person's weight and to send feedback to them. Similarly, wearable technology such as 'smart clothes' can be used to monitor heart rate.) This chapter describes the emerging area of e-health promotion, identifies the scope of this field, and discusses the opportunities and challenges that it presents.

In many developed countries e-health is being touted as one of the primary solutions to the challenges of twenty-first-century health care; specifically an ageing population living longer with chronic diseases which are increasingly expensive to treat. E-health is seen as providing the means to deliver more informed, empowered citizens who are better able to manage their own health; and to provide interventions for modifying lifestyle risk factors, all at low marginal cost using little in personnel resources. In England a review of the National Health Service (NHS) health informatics area has set out a vision where the public are empowered by having access to online health information, personalized 'wellness support,' and their own electronic health record (Department of Health 2008). The NHS has recently launched a website, NHS Choices (<http://www.nhs.uk>), which will carry general health advice as well as tools for delivering tailored, personalized health interventions.

The increasing availability and decreased cost of home broadband connections, the connected nature of the modern workplace, and a general increase in 'e-literacy' are helping to propel this revolution in online public health activity. In the UK in 2009 70% of households had internet access and 89% of UK adults had a mobile phone (Dutton *et al.* 2009). In developing countries mobile phone ownership is of increasing importance: in Africa mobile phones represent 90% of all telephone lines, and mobile-phone market penetration is at 30% (Lange 2009). Internet use via phones is increasing (Mobile Life 2008). The percentage of UK internet users using the internet to find information on health or medical care rose from 37% in 2005 to 68% in 2009 (Dutton *et al.* 2009). A US survey found that 61% of all adults reported using the internet for health information (Fox and Jones 2009).

The scope of e-health promotion

The internet and related technologies offer particular benefits for health-related activities. The convenience of 24-hour access from almost anywhere removes some of the traditional barriers to seeking help and to the delivery of health interventions. The privacy afforded by a personal device, coupled with the option of anonymity in most online activity, offers benefits for health promotion issues which may be stigmatizing (such as obesity or sexual behaviour). The scalability of most information-technology-based interventions generally gives them a very low marginal cost: once the intervention is developed it is relatively cheap to increase the delivery from a few users to millions. This also means that even a small health benefit may well be cost-effective. The geographical reach of the internet allows access to interventions across borders and cultures. Some examples illustrating the scope of e-health promotion activities are shown in Box 11.1.

The internet and other new technologies can be used as platforms for both mass-media approaches and for the delivery of individually targeted interventions. However, e-health is also offering new possibilities for health promotion, and some of the examples in Box 11.1 demonstrate this.

Box 11.1 The scope of e-health promotion activities

A stand-alone kiosk in a public area

There are a range of interactive health and wellbeing kiosks now available. Some give general health information and advice, whereas others cover specific issues. Some incorporate physiological measures such as weight, pulse, blood pressure, and oxygen saturation. In Hull, UK a scheme has used vending-machine-style kiosks which provide sexual health advice via a touch-screen interface, and which can also dispense condoms and chlamydia testing kits. They were aimed at young people and placed in community settings such as colleges, health centres, and supermarkets (<http://www.hullpct.nhs.uk/templates/page.aspx?id=4947>).

Internet intervention using website, e-mails, and text messaging

A randomized controlled trial (RCT) of a UK-based automated physical activity programme used multiple e-health tools to achieve a higher level of moderate physical activity in the intervention group (Hurling *et al.* 2007). A website tool helped participants to identify perceived barriers to physical activity, and offered solutions. Participants could report their level of physical activity each week through the website and receive constructive feedback. A physical activity planning tool used both e-mail and mobile-phone reminders to encourage participants to achieve their goals. There was also a web-based discussion board for participants to interact with each other. The outcome measures included 'real-time' collection of physical activity data using Bluetooth-enabled accelerometers.

A mobile-phone-based game to enhance HIV/AIDS awareness

The Freedom HIV/AIDS project in India has used four mobile-phone-based games targeted at users from a range of sociodemographic backgrounds to deliver educational messages about HIV/AIDS. Within 4 months of launching the games had been downloaded more than

Box 11.1 The scope of e-health promotion activities *(cont)*

10 million times (<http://www.freedomhivaids.in/FreedomHiv
Aids.htm>).

An internet viral marketing game to generate interest in a campaign

The Canadian Health Network used an internet-based viral marketing game to generate traffic to a health promotion website. An
initial distribution of a virtual running game to 200 hundred individuals was rapidly disseminated and reached over 100 000 within
15 days. Two-thirds of game participants completed at least one
educational health quiz. The Health Network experienced a significant increase in website traffic and subscribers to its newsletter
(Gosselin and Poitras 2008).

A website and e-mails to promote community action

An interactive website and an e-mail campaign were used by the
Calgary Tobacco Reduction Action Coalition, a group of health
workers and non-governmental organizations, to mobilize the
local community to advocate changes in a local smoking bylaw.
Users of the website received e-mail notifications of key events
related to the council decision process and how to contact their
councillors. The campaign appeared to influence the change in the
smoke-free bylaws and built local social capital (Grierson *et al.*
2006).

Initially e-health tools tended to mimic the social marketing campaigns and lifestyle interventions used in traditional settings, but
increasingly the producers of these tools are beginning to harness
their interactive and multimodal capability. As the e-health literacy of
both users and providers increases (Norman and Skinner 2006), the
potential of these tools to be personalized, flexible, and responsive is
being realized. By using information gathered from users over time,
tools can be targeted and tailored to the individual's situation, and
adapted as situations change. Interventions can be delivered across

multiple channels in a systematic, integrated manner. Interactivity means that outcomes can be measured, and feedback given, in real time. Physiological measurements, such as blood pressure, taken from personal digital monitoring devices can be incorporated, as can information from an individual's personal health record.

The effectiveness of e-health promotion

Much of the activity in e-health promotion has been focused on individual behaviour-change interventions using behavioural strategies. Certainly almost all the evidence supporting the use of e-health tools comes from this area. As a result there has been criticism that e-health researchers are taking a reductionist pre-Ottawa Charter approach to health promotion (de Leeuw 2008) (see Chapter 2 for further description of the historical context). However, perhaps a more likely and less conspiratorial explanation is that behavioural change tools can be readily evaluated using experimental study designs such as randomized trials (see Chapter 4), and such tools are often developed as commercial products which need to demonstrate some level of effectiveness prior to exploitation, providing a strong incentive for evaluation.

A Cochrane Collaboration review (see Chapter 6) of interactive health communication applications for chronic disease found improvements in knowledge, social support, health behaviours, and clinical outcomes, but they also noted variability across studies and called for larger, high-quality studies (Murray *et al.* 2005). A review of studies of web-based behavioural or health educational interventions which have had a non-web-based comparator as the control group found that many studies showed web-based interventions were superior in achieving knowledge or behaviour-change outcomes (Wantland *et al.* 2004). Recently several systematic reviews have examined the evidence of effectiveness for e-health behavioural-change interventions, mainly focused on dietary and physical activity interventions (Kroeze *et al.* 2006; Norman *et al.* 2007; van den Berg *et al.* 2007; Neville *et al.* 2009; Marcus *et al.* 2009). These reviews recognized that much of the evidence is of low methodological quality (see also Evers 2006), but found evidence that e-health interventions can be effective for dietary behaviour outcomes and for improving levels of physical activity. Many small studies have evaluated interventions for smoking cessation, showing that e-health tobacco interventions, mainly using websites or using mobile-phone text messaging, may be effective in improving quitting rates at short-term follow-up (Swartz *et al.* 2006; Free *et al.* 2009).

As an emerging area of study, and one that for the most part does not have the resources of the pharmaceutical industry behind it, the e-health literature has been dominated by relatively small studies of many pilot interventions, often with limited follow-up periods (Powell *et al.* 2005). The work so far clearly shows that such tools can be feasible, acceptable, and usable. But it is difficult to draw definitive conclusions regarding the effectiveness of e-health tools.

The opportunities and challenges of evaluation in e-health promotion

The methodological approaches recommended for use in e-health promotion are the same as for health promotion in general and should be based on the traditional tools of health services research. The UK Medical Research Council's complex interventions framework (Craig *et al.* 2008) (see Chapter 4) is useful because the majority of e-health promotion tools are multifaceted, complex interventions with various components which may not all be accessed by the user, and where it is not easy to disaggregate the active elements.

A key opportunity for e-health evaluators is to harness digital technology as a tool for doing the research as well as being the object under study. This is not only about saving resources, although that is clearly important, but as Murray *et al.* (2009) argue if one of the advantages of internet interventions is that they can capture people online who are not accessing other services, then we should evaluate this 'real-world' scenario as faithfully as possible (see Chapter 10, which discusses the scope for natural experiments). A good example of a pioneering study in this area is described in Box 11.2.

As the example in Box 11.2 demonstrates, participants in an e-health intervention study can be identified, recruited, and give consent to participate in the study online, with no need for contact between investigators and participants.

Box 11.2 Example of evaluation using an online randomized controlled trial

The Down Your Drink (DYD) protocol

This study, led by a team at University College London (Murray *et al.* 2007), is an excellent example of an online randomized controlled trial (RCT), exploiting the opportunities of e-research methods to evaluate an e-health tool. It was an interactive website intervention for excessive alcohol consumption which provided a structured 6 week programme based on the stages-of-change model, and including components of motivational enhancement, cognitive behavioural therapy, and relapse prevention. This was compared with a purely information-based website with no interactive components or structured programme. This study used e-methods from recruitment to final follow-up measures. Participants were recruited from internet users accessing the study website which is linked from a major charity website and from search engines. They completed an online screening test, and if eligible they completed an online consent form. Baseline measurements were taken online and automatic randomization then gave participants access to either the intervention or the control website. Use of the intervention was logged automatically on the web servers. Follow-up measures were collected using the study website and via e-mail. This was therefore a fully automated online RCT with no face-to-face contact between investigators and participants.

In the UK, ethics committees are beginning to accept internet-only consent without face-to-face contact, provided appropriate safeguards are in place. For example, in the Down Your Drink study featured in Box 11.2, the investigators required potential participants to read through the information sheets online before they indicated their consent by filling in an online form and also to provide an e-mail address which was then verified.

However, identity verification is a wider issue. In an online study, it is not only difficult to verify identity independently, but it is also hard to verify key personal characteristics such as age or gender. To verify identities would require participants to give out confidential personal information such as a National Insurance number which could be cross-checked, but this is likely to put off many potential participants. The culture of internet use is one of anonymity and, often, flexible identity. Visitors to chatrooms and bulletin boards use nicknames, and users are encouraged to never give out personal information. The investigators of e-health studies need to work with this culture and maximize their participation rates while providing no incentives to giving false information or to creating multiple identities. A compromise solution, used by many companies, is to require e-mail validation. This ensures that each participant holds a valid e-mail address and has accessed it to confirm their desire to participate. Participants can also be asked to provide their offline contact details, although there is no guarantee that genuine ones will be given (Murray *et al.* 2009).

In an online trial, collection of any self-reported baseline and follow-up measures can also be automated. However, self-report measures which have been validated for offline use, for example in a postal questionnaire, may not have been validated for use as an online assessment, where there may be slight differences in the psychometric properties (as it is difficult to exactly replicate the style and format) (Murray *et al.* 2009). The future is likely to see the wider use of networked personal devices which can provide physiological measurement (such as blood pressure), and these measures can also be incorporated into an e-trial. These e-research methods will bring benefits to many evaluations, not just those concerned with e-health interventions. There are also challenges around the legitimate uses of personal data, particularly as interventions become integrated with electronic health records, and in the issues of the security and confidentiality of these data.

Participant retention is a major issue in the experimental evaluation of e-health promotion tools. It is well established in the e-health literature that interventions suffer from high levels of participant attrition (Eysenbach 2005). There are often significant numbers of people who access e-health sites but who then either do not use the tool or use it in a limited way. Internet behaviour in general is often transitory and disjointed, and it is no surprise to find this with e-health interventions.

In terms of process evaluation, existing models and tools can be used for e-health interventions as for their offline counterparts. Examples include work by Evers and colleagues (2003) and by Skinner and colleagues (2006) who have both adapted models from traditional settings for use by e-health promotion (see Box 11.3).

Box 11.3 Process evaluation in e-health promotion

Evers and colleagues (2003) adapted an existing guideline for smoking cessation (the 5 'A' criteria provided by the US Public Health Service; Fiore *et al.* 2000) to create a tool for assessing whether internet behaviour-change programmes possess the minimum criteria to achieve change. These were described as: Advise—give advice to change; Assess—assessment of variables that may influence change such as willingness; Assist—providing assistance such as support and reinforcement; Anticipatory guidance—related to relapse prevention; and Arrange follow-up. They piloted their Health Behaviour Change on the Internet (HBC-I) tool on a sample of 273 websites across seven health behaviours. This study was conducted in 2003; they found that only 15% of websites met four or five of the criteria.

Skinner and colleagues (2006) developed their spiral technology action research (STAR) model, incorporating existing theories of behaviour change, action research, and quality improvement and showed how this had been used in the development of a youth smoking-prevention and -cessation website. The STAR model includes elements of software evaluation such as usability testing, and researchers such as Pagliari (2007) have argued for closer working between software developers and health service researchers to achieve better collaboration in e-health design and evaluation. Clearly there are differences between evaluating the functionality, usability, and acceptability of a piece of software, and its effectiveness as a tool for health promotion, but both assessments are required and can inform each other.

By their nature, e-health tools sit in an information-rich environment and tend to generate more potential process measures than offline interventions. Evaluators can collect detailed usage information not available in traditional settings. For example, web statistics can provide information on not only which pages of a website were accessed, but also at what time of day and for how long. Software can record whether links in e-mails are clicked on, or whether text messages are responded to, or how users entered and exited a website. If a tool requires some form of user authentication then evaluators are also able to identify who has accessed the site. Where users are not registered, software can give cookies to a user's browser so repeat visitors can be counted, even if not personally identified. However, some users choose to set their browser security settings to not accept cookies, so no software solution is perfect.

Increasingly e-health interventions are incorporating Web 2.0 social-networking elements and qualitative data from social exchanges can also be captured and analysed, subject to users having been informed and appropriate ethical approval given. This last point again touches on the challenge of the legitimate uses of personal data, and on the issues of the security and confidentiality of that data. Evaluators should follow an appropriate research governance framework and research participants should be informed as to how their data are being used.

Digital exclusion

Since the internet health care revolution started, academic and policy discourse has highlighted the issue of the digital divide (Korp 2006), and the inequalities between the 'have-nets' and the 'have-nots' (Powell *et al.* 2003). This has been the most consistent argument used against the introduction of e-health tools which may exclude those who do not have the equipment or skills to engage with new technologies. Certain groups may be excluded, and these may well be the same groups that suffer inequalities in a traditional (non-internet) health system. Likewise, groups that are already well served by existing systems may be further empowered and thus inequalities may widen.

Recently, we have seen a second digital divide occurring *within* the group who have adopted new technologies, due to differences in the capabilities of their equipment. For example the divide between those with broadband internet access compared with dial-up (Fox 2005), or between those with 3G smartphones and those with basic handsets. This second divide is important for interventions developed to exploit the latest platforms, or which depend on large amounts of data being transferred quickly.

Evaluators should collect sociodemographic data to examine the issue of digital exclusion and the internet. One study investigated the relationship between health-related internet use and various demographic variables in seven European countries (Andreassen *et al.* 2007). This work showed that health-related internet use was significantly related to younger age and to higher level of education attainment. This finding has been replicated in other studies (Powell and Clarke 2006). The European survey also found that women were more likely than men to use the internet for health-related reasons. People with long-term health problems or with a history of frequent visits to their general practitioner were also higher users of the internet, presumably reflecting greater health care need in these groups. The relationship with age is likely to be a cohort effect which will dissipate as the population ages and e-health literacy becomes more universal, but e-health developers and evaluators need to be aware that two important variables associated with ill health (namely old age and low level of education) are also associated with lower use of internet-based technologies.

Digital exclusion is less pronounced for mobile telephony and this has led to various attempts to harness the mobile phone as a tool for delivering health education to disadvantaged groups. Usage is fairly high across all socio-economic groups, but tails off in older age groups, especially in those aged over 75 (Ofcom 2008). Some evaluation studies have suggested that mobile-phone use may be higher in more deprived groups (e.g. Koivusilta *et al.* 2007) and while this is not a universal finding, evaluators should take note that mobile platforms may be more inclusive than platforms relying on home computer access.

The future

In high-income countries, the digital world is now becoming so integrated into daily life that there will no longer be a need for the term 'e-health'. Digital health care will become mainstream health care. In the near future the internet will become the main point of access for health services including the online booking of appointments, instant-messaging triage, the completion of pre-consultation questionnaires, checking of test results, accessing decision support tools, and the ordering of prescriptions. The development of the electronic health record into a personal record, owned by the patient, integrated with tailored health advice and decision-support tools, and accessed from home or mobile connections, will help to engage and empower individuals. The harnessing of Web 2.0 developments will see the provision of more health-related virtual communities to provide peer support to people with chronic illness and their carers. In the longer-term future, the near universality of mobile technology will make way for the ubiquity of pervasive technology where portable devices will be replaced by wearable and implantable devices. Health promotion interventions will be targeted, personalized, and delivered direct to the individual according to need, through 'always-on' connections, to 'always-there' devices.

In low- and middle-income countries, population rates of internet access are at relatively low levels, but mobile-phone markets are booming. While there is a relative lack of research evaluating e-health tools in this setting, promising findings are beginning to emerge (Vital Wave Consulting 2009). For example, in South Africa, Project Masiluleke sends over a million text messages a day written in local languages to encourage testing and treatment for HIV/AIDS. Text messaging has also been used to support tuberculosis treatment compliance. Both mobile phones and internet access are more likely to be shared between one or more individuals than in developed countries, and e-health providers need to be mindful of this.

In order to be economically sustainable, twenty-first-century health systems must shift their focus to the promotion of wellbeing, the prevention of ill health, and the early detection of illness. E-health tools and their integration across platforms, across sectors, and across the health professional/public divide can enable this transformational shift. Rigorous assessment of the effectiveness and cost-effectiveness of these new tools is essential, combined with evaluations of the organizational and cultural issues which promote or inhibit their use.

Key points

◆ E-health is the use of new information and communication technologies for improving health and health care.

◆ E-health tools can provide a cheap and effective way of avoiding some of the traditional barriers to help seeking and the delivery of health interventions.

◆ Much of the activity in e-health promotion has focussed on individual behaviour-change interventions which seek to modify lifestyle risk factors using behavioural strategies.

◆ The broad methodological approaches recommended for use in e-health promotion are the same as for health promotion in general, but e-health evaluation presents new opportunities and challenges, such as the ability to conduct whole trials online, and to collect new process measures.

◆ In the future digital health care will become mainstream health care.

References

Andreassen, H.K., Bujnowska-Fedak, M.M., Chronaki, C.E. *et al.* (2007) European citizens' use of E-health services: a study of seven countries. *BMC Public Health* **7**, 53.

Craig, P., Dieppe, P., Macintyre, S., Mitchie, S., Nazareth, I., and Petticrew, M. (2008) Developing and evaluating complex interventions: the new Medical Research Council guidance. *British Medical Journal* **337**, 979–83.

de Leeuw, E. (2008) Welcoming the e-age: the e-age has finally caught up with our Journal. *Health Promotion International* **23**, 207–8.

Department of Health (2008) *The Health Informatics Review Report.* http://www.dh.gov.uk/en/Publicationsandstatistics/Publications/PublicationsPolicyAndGuidance/DH_086073. Department of Health, London.

Dutton, W.H., Helsper, E.J., and Gerber, M.M. (2009) *Oxford Internet Survey 2009 Report: The Internet in Britain.* Oxford Internet Institute, Oxford.

Evers, K.E. (2006) Ehealth promotion: the use of the Internet for health promotion. *American Journal of Health Promotion* **20**, s1–7.

Evers, K.E., Prochaska, J.M., Prochaska, J.O., Driskell, M.M., Cummins, C.O., and Velicer, W.F. (2003) Strengths and weaknesses of health behavior change programs on the internet. *Journal of Health Psychology* **8**, 63–70.

Eysenbach, G. (2005) The law of attrition. *Journal of Medical Internet Research* **7**, e11.

Fiore, M.C., Bailey, W.C., Cohen, S.J. *et al.* (2000) *Treating Tobacco Use and Dependence (Clinical Practice Guideline).* US Department of Health and Human Services, Public Health Service, Rockville, MD.

Fox, S. (2005) *Digital Divisions.* Pew Internet and American Life Project, Washington DC.

Fox, S. and Jones, S. (2009) *The Social Life of Health Information.* Pew Internet and American Life Project, Washington DC.

Free, C., Whittaker, R., Knight, R., Abramsky, T., Rodgers, A., and Roberts, I.G. (2009). Txt2stop: a pilot randomised controlled trial of mobile phone-based smoking cessation support. *Tobacco Control* **18**, 88–91.

Gosselin, P. and Poitras, P. (2008) Use of an internet "viral" marketing software platform in health promotion. *Journal of Medical Internet Research* **10**, e47.

Grierson, T., van Dijk, M.W., Dozois, E., and Mascher, J. (2006) Using the Internet to build community capacity for healthy public policy. *Health Promotion Practice* **7**, 13–22.

Hurling, R., Catt, M., de Boni, M. *et al.* (2007) Using Internet and mobile phone technology to deliver an automated physical activity program: randomized controlled trial. *Journal of Medical Internet Research* **9**, e7.

Koivusilta, L.K., Lintonen, T.P., and Rimpela, A.H. (2007) Orientations in adolescent use of information and communication technology: a digital divide by sociodemographic background, educational career, and health. *Scandinavian Journal of Public Health* **35**, 95–103.

Korp, P. (2006) Health on the Internet: implications for health promotion. *Health Education Research* **21**, 78–86.

Kroeze, W., Werkman, A., and Brug, J. (2006) A systematic review of randomized trials on the effectiveness of computer-tailored education on physical activity and dietary behaviors. *Annals of Behavioral Medicine* **31**, 205–23.

Lange, P. (2009) *Africa – Mobile Market Growth Starting to Flatten.* www.telecomsmarketresearch.com/resources/Africa_overview.shtml.

Marcus, B.H., Ciccolo, J.T., and Sciamanna, C.N. (2009) Using electronic/computer interventions to promote physical activity. *British Journal of Sports Medicine* **43**, 102–5.

Mobile Life (2008) *The Connected World. Exploring our Relationships with Modern Technology in a Wireless World.* Mobile Life Report 2008. www.mobilelife2007.co.uk/Mobile_Life_2008.pdf. Carphone Warehouse and The London School of Economics and Political Science, London.

Murray, E., Burns, J., See Tai, S., Lai, R., and Nazareth, I. (2005) Interactive health communication applications for people with chronic disease. *Cochrane Database of Systematic Reviews* **4**, CD004274.

Murray, E., McCambridge, J., Khadjesari, Z. *et al.* (2007) The DYD-RCT protocol: an on-line randomised controlled trial of an interactive computer-based intervention compared with a standard information website to reduce alcohol consumption among hazardous drinkers. *BMC Public Health* **7**, 306.

Murray, E., Khadjesari, Z., White, I.R. *et al.* (2009) Methodological challenges in online trials. *Journal of Medical Internet Research* **11**, e9.

Neville, L.M., O'Hara, B., and Milat, A.J. (2009) Computer-tailored dietary behaviour change interventions: a systematic review. *Health Education Research* **24**, 699–720.

Norman, C.D. and Skinner, H.A. (2006) Ehealth literacy: essential skills for consumer health in a networked world. *Journal of Medical Internet Research* **8**, e9.

Norman, G.J., Zabinski, M.F., Adams, M.A., Rosenberg, D.E., Yaroch, A.L., and Atienza, A.A. (2007) A review of ehealth interventions for physical activity and dietary behavior change. *American Journal of Preventive Medicine* **33**, 336–45.

Ofcom (2008) *The Consumer Experience 2008. Research Report.* www.ofcom.org.uk/research/tce/ce08/research.pdf. Ofcom, London.

Pagliari, C. (2007) Design and evaluation in ehealth: challenges and implications for an interdisciplinary field. *Journal of Medical Internet Research* **9**, e15.

Powell, J. and Clarke, A. (2006) Internet information seeking in mental health: population survey. *British Journal of Psychiatry* **189**, 273–7.

Powell, J., Darvell, M., and Gray, J.A.M. (2003) The doctor, the patient and the world-wide web: how the internet is changing healthcare. *Journal of Royal Society of Medicine* **96**, 74–6.

Powell, J., Lowe, P., Griffiths, F.E., and Thorogood, M. (2005) A critical analysis of the literature on the internet and consumer health information. *Journal of Telemedicine and Telecare* **11**, s41–3.

Skinner, H.A., Maley, O., and Norman, C.D. (2006) Developing Internet-based Ehealth promotion programs: the spiral technology action research (STAR) model. *Health Promotion Practice* **7**, 406–17.

Swartz, L.H., Noell, J.W., Schroeder, S.W., and Ary, D.V. (2006) A randomised control study of a fully automated internet based smoking cessation programme. *Tobacco Control* **15**, 7–12.

van den Berg, M.H., Schoones, J.W., and Vliet Vlieland, T.P.M. (2007) Internet-based physical activity interventions: a systematic review of the literature. *Journal of Medical Internet Research* **9**, e26.

Vital Wave Consulting (2009) *mHealth for Development: The Opportunity of Mobile Technology for Healthcare in the Developing World.* UN Foundation-Vodafone Foundation Partnership, Washington DC.

Wantland, D.J., Portillo, C.J., Holzemer, W.L., Slaughter, R., and Mcghee, E.M. (2004) The effectiveness of Web-based vs. non-Web-based interventions: a meta-analysis of behavioral change outcomes. *Journal of Medical Internet Research* **6**, e40.

Part IV

Participants in, and users of, evaluation

Chapter 12

Involving lay people in the development of NICE public health guidance

Jane Cowl

The UK National Institute for Health and Clinical Excellence (NICE) provides guidance on promoting good health and preventing and treating ill health. NICE makes recommendations using the best available evidence. In 2005, the organization's remit widened from a clinical focus to include producing public health guidance on health promotion. As a result of this expanded remit, NICE began developing support for involving the public in public health guidance, building on the experience of involving lay people in our clinical guidance.

Public involvement in policy

Public bodies need to be responsive and accountable to the people they serve. Effective public involvement can contribute to more appropriate policies and services, where decision-making is informed by the experiences of the client group or community and what matters to them. National Health Service (NHS) organizations have a statutory duty to involve service users in the planning, development, and delivery of services (Department of Health 2008) and the NHS Constitution includes a user's right to involvement in health care and NHS decision-making (Department of Health 2009). NICE's commitment to involving the public in all its work is clear (NICE 2007). In line with its commitment to patient-centred *clinical* guidance, NICE aims to produce *public health* guidance which takes full account of issues that are important to the client group or wider community, by including evidence on their views and experiences and involving lay people in the decision-making process. It can be daunting for lay people working on expert committees, so staff in NICE's Patient and Public Involvement Programme are there to support the involvement of individuals and organizations that bring lay perspectives to the guidance-development process.

Opportunities for lay involvement

The main stages of work on public health guidance are outlined in Box 12.1. The following discussion focuses on the most developed stage for lay involvement, which is the process of guidance development.

Who to involve?

For public health topics, the challenge is that the relevant lay audience is much broader and less easily defined than it is for clinical topics (where the lay audience usually consists of patients, service users, carers, and organizations that represent their interests). Box 12.2 gives examples that illustrate the breadth of lay audiences for public health guidance.

Involving organizations that represent public interests

For each new guidance project, NICE identifies the organizations that represent public interests relevant to the topic and invites them to participate. National voluntary and non-governmental organizations (NGOs) and the Local Involvement Networks (LINks) can register as stakeholders for individual topics. (LINks were established in 2008 to give citizens a stronger voice in health and social care services.) Once registered, NICE automatically invites them to contribute at various stages of the guidance-development process. Staff in the Patient and Public Involvement team have found that personal contact has often proved fruitful in encouraging organizations to participate that would otherwise not have become involved.

As part of its commitment to transparency, NICE publishes on its website stakeholder comments on consultation documents along with responses from the guidance developers. For practical reasons NICE excludes local voluntary and community groups in this consultation process, but they are included when conducting fieldwork to test draft recommendations.

Box 12.1 Opportunities for lay involvement in public health guidance

Topic selection

Anyone can suggest a topic via the NICE website: <http://www.nice.org.uk/>. A Topic Consideration Panel, which includes three lay members, prioritizes suggestions.

Defining the scope of each guidance topic

NICE consults stakeholder organizations on the draft 'scope' which sets out what the guidance will and will not cover. Organizations representing public interests can influence the nature and direction of the guidance by contributing to this consultation process.

Development of guidance

Independent advisory groups consider the evidence and develop recommendations. There are at least three lay members per group. Advisory groups co-opt additional people and invite experts to give testimony, as required.

Testing out draft guidance

- **Consulting stakeholders on the draft guidance** This is an opportunity for organizations representing a client group or wider public interests to raise issues of concern.
- **Fieldwork** Draft recommendations are tested out with practitioners including people working for voluntary and community organizations. NICE is developing its approach to consulting members of the client group; for example, NICE has tested out draft recommendations with vulnerable young people who are potential beneficiaries of the guidance.

Publicizing and putting the guidance into practice

Lay people who have been involved in the development of public health guidance often play a role in its launch and other promotional activities. NICE also encourages organizations to promote NICE guidance and to use it to support their own activities.

Box 12.2 Examples of lay audiences for public health guidance

NICE has a series of workplace health promotion guidance (promoting mental wellbeing, physical activity, and smoking cessation). The potential beneficiaries who might be represented in guidance include a large section of the population.

NICE produced guidance on needle and syringe provision, for which the immediate audience is injecting drug users but the views and experiences of the wider community are also relevant, because the programmes need to operate successfully within community settings.

NICE does not vet organizations or exclude them because of their views, which means that pressure groups and organizations with opposing views can take part. For example, for guidance on workplace interventions to promote smoking cessation, NICE invited both pro- and anti-smoking campaign groups to become registered stakeholders.

Lay membership of groups developing public health guidance

NICE guidance is developed by independent advisory committees including public health and other relevant professionals and researchers. Each committee has at least three lay members. Box 12.3 shows an example of the lay membership of a committee developing guidance on the prevention of alcohol-related disorders. Members of guidance development committees consider the evidence and develop recommendations and all members have equal status. The intention in involving lay people at this level of 'collaboration' is that they will ensure that community views inform the guidance's development and its recommendations (Involve 2005).

The time commitment expected from lay members is substantial and in recognition of the value of lay involvement NICE pays these members a fee as well as reimbursing expenses. The NICE Patient and Public Involvement Programme provide these members with dedicated

Box 12.3 Lay membership of the group developing guidance on prevention of alcohol-use disorders

1. Officer of a national charity working with and for families affected by substance misuse

2. Someone with personal and family experience of alcohol problems and member of a local service-user organization

3. Member of voluntary sector health promotion provider and former health officer for a minority ethnic umbrella organization

4. Trustee and former director of an inner-city charity working with individuals and communities with problems caused by alcohol misuse

information, training, and ongoing support. Training for lay members includes: sessions on the research methods used in developing guidance, with exercises in critical appraisal; consideration of health inequalities; and the opportunity for participants to explore their role and share experiences.

In addition to lay committee members, other community or service-user advocates may be invited to meetings to help committees understand more about the experiences of the client groups. They may join the advisory group as co-optees to work alongside the other members, or be invited to a specific meeting to give testimony as experts. For example, two lay people with wide networks and knowledge of needle and syringe programmes gave testimony to the Public Health Interventions Advisory Committee. Their up-to-date contributions from a client perspective included information not available in the research evidence and added value to the development of the needle and syringe programme guidance.

Recruiting lay people

NICE aims to recruit lay people who have the confidence and ability to contribute client or community perspectives within the context of a scientific process. This involves using a transparent recruitment process with an explicit role description and person specification, and advertising the vacancies on NICE's website and through stakeholder networks.

'Representativeness' is not relevant or achievable in the relatively small number of people sitting on an advisory body. This applies to both professionals and lay members of the group. Instead, NICE seeks to recruit lay members for their individual experience and expertise, which is informed by their community networks. Lay members are not required to act as a representative of an organization or group but to draw on their own understanding of community and equality issues and the research evidence.

Incorporating lay views and experiences

Sometimes guidance groups feel they need more information on user or community views and experiences than is available in the literature. They may use evidence from the testimony of community or service-user advocates. For some topics NICE has worked with other agencies to conduct small-scale consultation with members of a client group, and these findings have contributed to the development of the guidance or the validation of draft recommendations. Occasionally NICE may commission primary research to fill a major gap in evidence on the views and experiences of the client group (see Box 12.4).

Evaluation of lay involvement in guidance development

In the process of supporting lay participants in NICE's public health work, staff in the Patient and Public Involvement team receive informal feedback on what is working well and act on any problems that need addressing. Written feedback is also sought from participants at the training days for lay members of advisory groups. Informally NICE have received positive examples of the impact of lay involvement in public health work, both from lay people themselves and other committee members and observers. NICE is currently completing a formal evaluation using semi-structured questionnaires with former lay members and chairs of groups that have produced public health guidance. A report will be available in 2010.

Box 12.4 Preventing the uptake of smoking by children and young people

Gaps in the evidence on young people's perspectives on this topic were identified. The issues were twofold: young people's use of new media and raising the legal age for buying cigarettes from age 16 to 18. NICE commissioned qualitative research with young people to find out their views and experiences in relation to these issues. Focus groups that achieved the required diversity in terms of age, gender, and smoking status, and included young people excluded from school, were used. The findings demonstrated that young people regularly access a range of media sources which may all provide suitable means of delivering health promotion messages. Participants did not feel that the change in the law would be effective in preventing or stopping smoking among under 18s, although about half of the non-smokers felt that the law may make access difficult. A report of the full findings helped inform the development of the guidance (National Collaborating Centre for Drug Prevention 2008).

A previous study of lay involvement in developing clinical guidelines (NICE 2004) showed that the majority of lay respondents and chairs felt that the patient voice was heard and reflected in the guidelines. Most lay respondents rated their overall experience as a member of the group very positively; 13 of the 14 chairs rated it as 'excellent' or 'good', and all chairs who were interviewed thought the lay members had made contributions to the guidelines. However, both lay respondents and chairs identified specific areas for improving the experience of lay members and the effectiveness of their contributions. These included chairing of meetings and providing training and support.

The key role of the chair

Skilled chairs are fundamental to the success of the group and lay members' integration. Lay respondents, who spoke favourably about a chair's ability to facilitate the meetings, also felt well supported.

The importance of training and support

Training and support has developed over time in response to feedback. Some lay respondents thought that it would be good to hear first hand what to expect when they begin their work. As a result, training now routinely includes contributions from former lay members, and these sessions are highly valued. Another innovation is a follow-up workshop for lay people who are at least 6 months into their work with NICE. This was a response to requests from new recruits for an opportunity to share experiences and reflect on issues arising further down the line.

In summary, NICE has developed mechanisms for involving the public in its work and supporting that involvement for mutual benefit. The Key points box provides a checklist for developing a successful involvement strategy and reflects key aspects of the experience at NICE. In the development of public health guidance NICE aims to incorporate the perspectives of client groups so that the final recommendations are acceptable and appropriate to them. We will continue to refine our approach in response to lessons learned.

Key points

- To ensure effective involvement it is essential to first have both corporate commitment to, and a clear policy on, public involvement.
- The organization's policy on public involvement should consider issues of remuneration of lay people.
- If vulnerable groups are to be involved then appropriate arrangements should be made to make their involvement possible.
- It is important to be clear what input is needed from the public. This should be decided in consultation with public stakeholders.
- The process of identifying who to involve will take time and is a crucial step.

- Staff capacity and expertise are needed to support involvement work.
- There is a need to evaluate public involvement activities in order to revise and improve the process.

References

Department of Health (2008) *Real Involvement: Working with People to Improve Health Services.* <http://www.dh.gov.uk/en/Publicationsandstatistics/Publications/PublicationsPolicyAndGuidance/DH_089787>. Department of Health, London.

Department of Health (2009) *The NHS Constitution: The NHS Belongs To Us All.* <http://www.dh.gov.uk/en/Healthcare/NHSConstitution/index.htm>. Department of Health, London.

Involve (2005) *People and Participation.* <http://www.involve.org.uk/people_and_participation/>.

National Collaborating Centre for Drug Prevention (2008) *The Prevention of Uptake of Smoking by Children and Young People, with Reference to the Areas of Mass Media and the Sale of Tobacco Products: Findings from a Multi-method Primary Research Study. Final Report.* <http://www.nice.org.uk/nicemedia/pdf/PH14focusgroupreport.pdf>. National Collaborating Centre for Drug Prevention at Liverpool John Moores University Centre for Public Health, Liverpool.

NICE (2004) *A Report on a Study to Evaluate Patient/Carer Membership of the First NICE Guideline Development Groups.* <http://www.nice.org.uk/getinvolved/patientandpublicinvolvement/patientandpublicinvolvementprogramme/a_report_on_a_study_to_evaluate_patient_carer_membership_of_the_first_nice_guideline_development_groups.jsp>. National Institute for Health and Clinical Excellence, London.

NICE (2007) *Patient, Carer and Public Involvement Policy.* <http://www.nice.org.uk/getinvolved/patientandpublicinvolvement/patientandpublicinvolvementpolicy/patient_and_public_involvement_policy.jsp>. National Institute for Health and Clinical Excellence, London.

Chapter 13

Evaluating the ethics of health promotion: understanding informed participation

Dalya Marks

Ethical issues in health promotion are often overlooked. Interventions are planned, executed, and evaluated with little regard to ethical concerns. There is an assumption that health promotion is good for you and compliance is expected. This chapter examines some of the issues surrounding participation in health promotion interventions and considers what is required to acquire informed consent and promote informed decision-making.

Informed consent requires that participants are provided with unbiased information on the risks and benefits of an intervention, and are free to decide whether or not to take part. In addition to practical problems in delivering the information, acquiring informed consent might create conflict between health professionals' desire to achieve a high programme uptake while accepting that an informed person might decide *not* to participate. This chapter will suggest that in evaluating a health promotion programme outcomes should not be measured simply in terms of uptake, but *informed* uptake. Evaluation should include measures of knowledge and empowerment, not simply acceptance or refusal.

Current guidelines

The UK General Medical Council (GMC) guidelines for seeking patients' consent (see Box 13.1) do not state how much information

Box 13.1 Guidelines on informed consent for screening procedures

The following should be explained before the test:

+ the purpose of screening,
+ the likelihood of receiving a positive or negative result,
+ the chance of a false-positive or false-negative result,
+ the risks and uncertainties of the process,
+ the potential for financial and/or social discrimination.

The following should be explained after the test:

+ follow-up plans,
+ availability of support or counselling services.

General Medical Council (1999).

should be given or how it should be conveyed to facilitate informed decision-making.

The UK National Screening Committee guidelines (Department of Health 2000) state:

> There is a responsibility to ensure that those who accept an invitation (to screening) do so on the basis of informed choice, and appreciate that in accepting an invitation or participating in a programme to reduce their risk of a disease there is a risk of an adverse outcome.

Informed choice implies that a decision to refuse a test or an invitation to participate is as valid an outcome as acceptance.

Participant involvement in decision-making

An individual should be able to make an informed choice about whether to participate or not, through provision of the necessary information about the benefits *and* disadvantages of such a decision (Department of Health 2000; Jepson *et al.* 2000). This process has been described as:

> a reasoned choice. . .made by a reasonable individual using relevant information about the advantages and disadvantages of all the possible courses of action, in accord with the individual's beliefs.

(Bekker *et al.* 1999)

Whether this adequately describes what is experienced is unclear. Although it corresponds well with respect for autonomy, little is known about the effectiveness of involving patients in decisions about their care, or the effect that sharing information will have (Entwistle *et al.* 1998).

Informed choice requires a discussion to take place between a participant and the health professional promoting the 'informed' aspect. There is a continuum of where the responsibility for that decision takes place, with shared decision-making (SDM) at one end and informed decision-making at the other. SDM involves at least two parties (the client and the professional) and both have to reach consensus (Whelan *et al.* 1997). SDM recognizes the importance of participant preference but includes a role for the health professional who is equipped with the technical knowledge, whereas informed decision-making assumes that the participant will make the decision alone (Coulter 1997). With SDM, both the process of the decision-making and the outcome (intervention choice) are shared, requiring joint access to the evidence supporting decisions rather than an abdication of professional responsibility (Coulter 1997). Some commentators caution that SDM cannot bear the entire burden for informing and involving individuals and that population-orientated interventions promoting informed decision-making should be explored (Briss *et al.* 2004).

The introduction of participant involvement in decision-making has led to tensions between traditionalists and those advocating individual choice. Traditionalists fear that the promotion of individual choice may endanger the goal of improving the public's health. For example, in the UK, following a media-led scare about the safety of the combined measles, mumps, and rubella vaccination, many parents chose not to immunize their children. As a result, the proportion of children immunized fell to dangerous levels, and there is now concern about both measles and mumps epidemics. However, individual decision-making need *not* be incompatible with broader public interest or 'communitarian' values if the shift in power or decision-making from professional to patient incorporates autonomy, rights, and responsibilities (Parker 2001).

The tension between respecting individual autonomy while trying to maximize the benefits for the population has been discussed with reference to a population cardiovascular screening programme (Marteau *et al.* 2002). The programme aimed to reduce population-level morbidity and mortality, and the information provided was brief, highlighting the health benefits of participation while neglecting the potential harms. These 'harms' could be the identification of one's susceptibility to coronary heart disease, which would require long-term monitoring, adherence to medication, and/or lifestyle changes. The authors argue that attendance might be reduced if a more balanced account of the implications of participation is provided. However, if those participating are more motivated to adopt the recommendations, the longer-term outcomes could be more favourable, and the programme might be more cost-effective.

Problems with delivery

Little is known about the effects of providing patients with a full account of the risks and benefits of the intervention they have been offered. Not only do we not know how best to provide this information, we know even less about the effect of providing informed decision-making in terms of uptake (Jepson *et al.* 2000). Information may increase knowledge about the intervention, but not acceptability, as was found in a study of parental acceptance of human papillomavirus (HPV) screening (see Box 13.2) (Dempsey *et al.* 2006). It is assumed that the more a person knows about the condition and the impact of the intervention, the less the psychological distress will be, but this is not supported by evidence.

The ability of the target audience to absorb the information is important. Data from a study assessing the readability of patient information leaflets in general practice estimate that 5.5 million people in the UK have reading difficulties and 22% of the working population have low literacy levels (Smith *et al.* 1998). This issue is even more important in low-income countries where literacy levels are lower.

The focus of patient information leaflets tends to be on presentation and readability rather than content, which can lead to inaccurate and misleading information, based on unscientific clinical opinion (Coulter 1998). The basic ground rules of effective communication include the exchange of accurate information, exploration of anxieties

Box 13.2 Human papillomavirus vaccination programme in schools

Thirteen-year-old girls in the UK are being immunized against human papillomavirus (HPV), which causes cervical cancer, through a school-based programme. Because they are aged under 16, consent is required from a parent or guardian. This might result in discord between the young person and parent. The vast majority of research in this area has focused on factors relating to parental attitudes and consent, rather than the young people's views.

Young people aged under 16 can attend a confidential sexual health clinic and access a range of services without parental consent, yet parental consent is required for the girl to have the HPV vaccine. A third of parents who were asked their views about the child's right to consent to HPV vaccination within a sexual-health setting without parental consent insisted that they still be involved in the decision-making process (Brabin *et al.* 2007). If consent procedures differ from one setting to another, there is the potential for friction within the family unit as parental rights are upheld over those of the adolescents.

or concerns, opportunities for expressing empathy, awareness of treatment options, and a negotiation of different views.

Problems can arise if the information presented is not tailored to individuals' needs, beliefs, and values, but rather have a one-size-fits-all approach (Goyder *et al.* 2000). If individuals' values and competing priorities are not taken into account, both participants and health professionals may be faced with conflicting demands.

Newer technologies such as interactive CD-ROMs, computer decision tools, or the internet may focus attention further onto appearance rather than substance. Few such technological decision aids have been evaluated, but it appears that they can improve knowledge and realistic expectations, enhance active participation in decision-making, and improve agreement between choice and values (O'Connor *et al.* 2003). It may be that such advances in communication lead to greater highlighting of the uncertainties around medical interventions or outcomes, which in turn may make decisions harder to make. A review of the evidence on presenting risk information has suggested that when patients receive information that is more understandable they become increasingly cautious in deciding whether to accept treatment, comply with interventions or participate in trials (Edwards *et al.* 2001). Even when stringent consent processes are present, and information is provided orally and in writing, there may still be a discrepancy between a health professional's account and a lay person's understanding of the nature of the condition being screened for (see Box 13.3).

Box 13.3 Screening for familial hypercholesterolaemia: an example of misunderstanding

A qualitative study (Marks 2004) of 20 relatives of individuals with familial hypercholesterolaemia (FH; a condition which carries a high risk of premature heart disease) found that despite following a carefully established protocol, with a high participation rate, there was still much misunderstanding and confusion after participants had been screened. Understanding of the condition, risk of transmission to self and family, and what lifestyle modifications were effective differed greatly from the information that the nurse thought had been provided.

It cannot be assumed that, just because information is provided and formal consent procedures are undertaken, people will act in the expected way. Some of the participants who tested negative for FH were left with heightened awareness of their disease risk and lingering fears about whether they were still at risk of developing heart disease. Participation in this screening programme did not allay concerns about disease susceptibility.

This research, using qualitative methods, demonstrated unanticipated effects that had not been considered previously. Regrettably, qualitative research is not often incorporated into programme evaluations or assessments of social 'costs' in cost-effectiveness analyses.

Informed participation: potential tensions

The tension between individual choice, autonomy, and what is considered to be in a participant's best interests is frequently raised. For example, a participant might be well informed (presented with the benefits and risks) and then may make a decision which the clinician or health professional feels is not the right one, but this decision might be appropriate for the participant (Ashcroft *et al.* 2001). Decisions are made within the context of one's environment, and this complex interaction must be understood and respected when one course of action is chosen over another. Sometimes a decision not to undergo further tests might be appropriate, and thus the choice *not* to present for screening should be accepted as a positive outcome if the objective of the programme is to encourage *informed* uptake.

A systematic review (see Chapter 6) explored the concept of informed uptake, examining factors associated with participation, and assessing the effectiveness of methods to increase uptake in screening programmes (Jepson *et al.* 2000). The authors found limited evidence on how providing information affects uptake. Only four of the 190 intervention studies reported giving information on the risks and benefits, and only one study evaluated the effect of this knowledge on the decision-making process. Evidence was inconclusive on how different types of information might affect screening knowledge or uptake. This review concluded that when trying to increase participation, knowledge should be measured as an outcome in the decision-making process, and that future studies should evaluate both informed uptake and actual uptake. Giving a balanced account might result in refusal to participate, which the health professional may not feel is a sensible choice, but it will have to be accepted as a valid outcome.

Uncertainty still exists about what is the most effective method to convey information to individuals, but there is agreement that adequate information should be provided.

In evaluating health promotion interventions, ethical aspects including the acquisition of consent should be considered; informed participation as well as actual uptake should be evaluated. Individuals make decisions based on their own beliefs and values, as well as their own perception of the risks involved. If an individual makes an informed decision not to participate, it should be regarded as an appropriate decision.

Key points

♦ Individuals have the right to expect a full explanation of the risks and benefits of an intervention before consenting to participate.

♦ People have the right to make an informed decision *not* to participate.

♦ If, after assessing the information, a decision not to participate is made, that needs to be valued.

♦ In evaluating health promotion interventions, informed uptake rather than throughput should be measured.

References

Ashcroft, R., Hope, T., and Parker, M. (2001) Ethical issues and evidence-based patient choice. In A. Edwards and G. Elwyn, eds, *Evidence-based Patient Choice: Inevitable or Impossible?*, pp. 53–65. Oxford University Press, Oxford.

Bekker, H., Thornton, J.G., Airey, C.M. *et al.* (1999) Informed decision making: an annotated bibliography and systematic review. *Health Technology Assessment* **3**(1), 1–156.

Brabin, L., Roberts, S.A., and Kitchener, H.C. (2007) A semi-qualitative study of attitudes to vaccinating adolescents against human papillomavirus without parental consent. *BMC Public Health* **7**, 20.

Briss, P.R., Reilley, B., Coates, R. *et al.* (2004) Promoting informed decisions about cancer screening in communities and healthcare systems. *American Journal of Preventive Medicine* **26**(1), 67–80.

Coulter, A. (1997) Partnerships with patients: the pros and cons of shared clinical decision-making. *Journal of Health Services Research and Policy* **2**(2), 112–21.

Coulter, A. (1998) Evidence based patient information is important, so there needs to be a national strategy to ensure it. *British Medical Journal* **317**, 225–6.

Dempsey, A.F., Zimet, G.D., Davis, R.L., and Koutsky, L. (2006) Factors that are associated with parental acceptance of human papillomavirus vaccines: a randomized intervention study of written information about HPV. *Pediatrics* **117**(5), 1486–93.

Department of Health (2000) Second Report of the National Screening Committee.

Edwards, A., Elwyn, G., Covey, J., Matthews, E., and Pill, R. (2001) Presenting risk information-a review of the effects of 'framing' and other manipulations on patient outcomes. *Journal of Health Communication* **6**, 61–82.

Entwistle, V.A., Sheldon, T.A., Sowden, A., and Watt, I.S. (1998) Evidence-informed patient choice. Practical issues of involving patients in decisions about health care technologies. *International Journal of Technology Assessment in Health Care* **14**(2), 212–25.

General Medical Council (1999) *Seeking Patients' Consent: the Ethical Considerations*. General Medical Council, London.

Goyder, E., Barratt, A., and Irwig, L.M. (2000) Telling people about screening programmes and screening test results: how can we do it better? *Journal of Medical Screening* **7**, 123–6.

Jepson, R., Clegg, A., Forbes, C., Lewis, R., Sowden, A., and Kleijnen, J. (2000) The determinants of screening uptake and interventions for increasing uptake: a systematic review. *Health Technology Assessment* **14**(14), 1–123.

Marks, D. (2004) *An evaluation of strategies for detecting familial hypercholesterolaemia. Public Health and Policy*. PhD thesis, University of London, London.

Marteau, T.M. and Kinmouth, A.L. (2002) Screening for cardiovascular risk: public health imperative or matter for individual informed choice? *British Medical Journal* **325**, 78–81.

O'Connor, A., Stacey, D., Entwistle, V. *et al.* (2003) Decision aids for people facing health treatment or screening decisions. *Cochrane Database of Systematic Reviews* **2**, CD001431 [update of Cochrane Database of Systematic Reviews (2001) 3, CD001431].

Parker, M. (2001) The ethics of evidence-based patient choice. *Health Expectations* **4**(2), 87–91.

Smith, H., Gooding, S., Brown, R., and Frew, A. (1998) Evaluation of readability and accuracy of information leaflets in general practice for patients with asthma. *British Medical Journal* **317**, 264–5.

Whelan, T., Gafni, A., and Charles, C. (1997) Shared decision-making in the medical encounter: what does it mean? (or it takes at least two to tango). *Social Science and Medicine* **44**(5), 681–92.

Chapter 14

Feeding back evaluation results to stakeholder participants

Yolande Coombes

In its simplest terms, feedback is defined as the information about the result of an experiment or the modification of a process by its result (*Oxford English Dictionary*). Therefore it might be said that evaluation is feedback. Learning from what we have done and incorporating those lessons to improve our interventions are the reasons why we evaluate. All too often, the results of an evaluation are not fed back to all those who have a stake in the programme or project. This chapter looks at the importance of disseminating research and evaluation results back to *all* participants in a project and focuses on the benefits of feedback to stakeholder participants from an ethical viewpoint, and to promote more effective implementation. It analyses the motivational effects of evaluation data being fed back to project implementers illustrated through a case study of feedback to antenatal care providers in Malawi.

The stakeholders for feedback

All projects have multiple stakeholders. A stakeholder is any person or group with an interest in the project being evaluated or in the results of the evaluation. It is possible to divide stakeholders into two distinct categories: stakeholder decision-makers and stakeholder participants. Box 14.1 indicates the types of stakeholder in the two broad categories.

There is a tendency for the focus to be on the dissemination of results to stakeholder decision-makers. It makes perfect sense that those who have funded an intervention or project should receive the

Box 14.1 Categories of stakeholder

Stakeholder decision-makers

- Funders and donors
- Policy-makers
- Researchers and academic community

Stakeholder participants

- Project staff and implementers
- Community leaders, community organizations, and interest groups
- Project participants or clients

results of an evaluation. Likewise, no one would disagree that results of health promotion interventions must be disseminated back to policy-makers, and to researchers to improve the evidence base for health promotion (see Chapter 15 for a more detailed discussion on getting results into policy). However, projects that only feed back to stakeholder decision-makers miss opportunities for promoting health and having a more immediate effect on health outcomes by focusing feedback to stakeholder participants.

Feedback to stakeholder decision-makers

This feedback 'upwards' tends to be a slow and cumbersome process. Researchers usually focus on publishing results in academic journals, and even with 'fast-track' systems they may not be in the public domain for a year. Another lag follows before they are combined with other research results to form policy. Balas and Boren (2000) found that it takes 17 years to turn only 14% of original research to the benefit of patient care. Furthermore, minority groups and the underserved usually gain access to effective interventions even more slowly. Evidence-based health promotion is vital for decision-making. However, we also have an ethical duty to patients and practitioners to get information back to them quickly, to assist them with their own decision-making.

Glasgow *et al.* (2003) argue that the reason for the slow and uneven translation of research findings into practice in the health promotion sciences is the lack of attention to issues of generalization and external validity (moderating factors that potentially limit the robustness of interventions). There needs to be greater understanding of, and research on, contextual factors. It is important to know that not only is a programme effective but that it is effective in other settings (see Chapters 4, 5, and 10 for discussions of internal and external validity).

Steckler and McLeroy (2008) noted that researchers tend to focus on maximizing internal validity to demonstrate whether a given health promotion intervention works under highly controlled conditions rather than to know if it will work among different population groups, organizations or settings (external validity). They criticize funding organizations and journals (stakeholder decision-makers) for being more concerned with the scientific rigor of interventions than the generalizability of results, and conclude that the emphasis on internal validity has contributed to the failure to translate research into practice in a timely manner.

Since evaluations are often carried out by an external agency or academic unit, the project staff participants and community (stakeholder participants) may or may not get to see the results. Even if they do they may not be in an appropriate format for them to use so that they can make the necessary changes to their practice or to their health.

Feedback to stakeholder participants

Feedback to all stakeholders including those who participated, either as practitioners or as users, or who stand to benefit (for example community groups) should be seen as a fundamental component of any evaluation. There are three main reasons to feedback to stakeholder participants: the first is an ethical obligation, the second is to improve the intervention, and the final reason is to validate the results.

Ethical obligation

As health promotion involves working to intrinsically improve people's health it requires a series of value judgements about what improved health is, and how we should intervene to obtain it.

There are four widely accepted ethical principles (Beauchamp and Childress 1989):

+ respect for autonomy (the rights of individuals to determine their lives);
+ beneficence (doing good);
+ non-maleficence (doing no harm);
+ justice (being fair and equitable).

It is likely that any intervention will touch on at least one of these ethical principles if not all of them. It is not unethical for an intervention to be found to be going against one of the ethical principles during an evaluation; but it is unethical not to tell the stakeholder participants once those results are known. For example, two randomized controlled trials on male circumcision as an HIV-prevention intervention were stopped because the lower rate of HIV in the circumcised group was so great it was ethically not possible to continue, and the intervention had to be offered to all groups as quickly as possible (WHO/UNAIDS 2007).

Improving the intervention

Whereas evaluation findings must be reported objectively, interpreting those findings and reaching conclusions can be a challenging process. Evaluators should include key stakeholder participants in this process by reviewing findings and preliminary conclusions with them prior to writing a formal report. Circulating an interim report and meeting to discuss it provides a means of obtaining feedback on the evaluation. Discussions with staff can provide new perspectives on the meaning and interpretation of the findings. These perspectives can then be included in the final report. An interim evaluation can be used to change the intervention and re-evaluate those changes before the end of the project. This is far more useful than waiting for a final evaluation once the project (and funding) has ended. For example, a mid-term review of a Marie Stopes social franchising project funded by KFW (Kreditan fur Wiederaufbau) in Kenya identified that the project was not meeting its targets for the outcome: couple years of protection (CYPs). The intervention was reorganized and problems addressed so that by the end of the first phase of funding the project had exceeded the target for CYPs. The mid-term evaluation can be essential for making corrections to the project design as flaws show up in implementation. Timely corrections increase the chances of project success (Marie Stopes International 2007).

It is not only important to involve stakeholder participants who are implementing but also those who are the users or clients because this can have an effect on their participation, compliance, and the ultimate success of a project. Green and Mercer (2001) assert that there is 'Ample evidence that disseminating the results of studies and telling people how they should incorporate this information into their lives produces minimal behaviour change.' They suggest that involving participants more in research and evaluation is a promising alternative to top-down assistance from experts and may help to ensure that evaluation results address real needs and will be used.

Strengthening external validity

Involving all stakeholders in both the evaluation and dissemination of results may help to ensure that the evaluation process goes more smoothly but more importantly the feedback from participants on the results presented to them can also become part of the intervention and enhance understanding of the external validity.

Understanding the experience of the intervention from the participant stakeholder's perspective is an important element of process evaluation (see Chapter 7). Combined with the points made above on ethical obligation and using feedback to improve the evaluation, feedback dialogue is an essential tool within an evaluation to understand the setting, and to understand how the intervention was carried out on the ground, in addition to how it was received and perceived. Interpreting this information accurately is indispensable for extending an intervention to population scale.

When results can be fed back to stakeholder participants, the process of feedback meets ethical obligations, and provides another learning opportunity to understand the barriers and facilitating factors, which will in turn aid our understanding of the external validity of the intervention. In addition it provides practitioners with evidence to make immediate changes.

How to feed back to participant stakeholders

Disseminating the evaluation findings is a critical step in building support for a programme. Evaluators should plan the process carefully and build in opportunities to share findings with stakeholder participants prior to the final report so the participants have an opportunity to contribute before it is completed. It is important to use appropriate methods of dissemination. In their analysis of systematic reviews of dissemination strategies and implementation of research Bero *et al.* (1998) concluded that passive dissemination is generally ineffective and that it is necessary to use specific strategies to encourage implementation of research-based recommendations to ensure changes in practice. Similarly, Brownson *et al.* (2007) call for more innovative approaches to dissemination which are more active with better adaptation to the range of audience. It is important that feedback to stakeholder participants is appropriate in style and language, using different strategies such as local media, face-to-face feedback, individual written reports, and community dialogue.

The case study in Box 14.2 shows that although Malawi had introduced an evidence-based policy for presumptive intermittent treatment of sulphadoxine-pyrimethamine (PIT-SP), in practice this policy was not being followed. Feedback from the evaluation which promoted practice guidelines improved the effectiveness of the policy. Feedback to participant stakeholders in the clinics took the form of a discussion with clinic staff and hands-on arrangement of the clinic infrastructure so that directly observed treatment could be introduced. Showing staff where they were relative to the other clinics was very motivating and helped them to unite as a team. Finally information, education, and communication materials specifically for pregnant women addressed some of the knowledge gaps and concerns they had.

The changes in increased sulphadoxine-pyrimethamine uptake took place in less than 6 months. Conversely, it took 12 months to get this study written up and published (Ashwood-Smith *et al.* 2002), and longer for the policy to be rewritten. In countries with endemic malaria such as Malawi, malaria during pregnancy can lead to maternal anaemia, low birth weight, and foetal death. These effects are compounded among primigravidae (of whom almost half will be parasitaemic at first

Box 14.2 Case study. Feeding back results to antenatal clinic staff and patients in Malawi

Presumptive intermittent treatment (PIT) for malaria in pregnancy is a proven method of reducing morbidity and mortality. In Malawi a policy on PIT using two doses of sulphadoxine-pyrimethamine (SP) was introduced in 1993. Initial research suggested the policy was not being followed; few women were receiving two doses of PIT-SP. An evaluation in Blantyre District, jointly undertaken by the Blantyre Integrated Malaria Initiative and the Malawi Safe Motherhood project, identified factors affecting PIT-SP rates (Coombes *et al.* 2003).

The evaluation consisted of: interviews with health staff and pregnant women attending antenatal clinics; review of antenatal patient records; and stock checks to assess SP availability and supply. The evaluation found that although 11 out of 12 facilities had adequate stocks of SP, only 44% of women received two doses of SP. In clinics which followed directly observed therapy (women taking the tablets at the clinic) a much higher rate of women got two doses. Staff were confused about the wording of the policy and the timing of the doses. The guidelines stated that the second PIT-SP dose should be given between 28 and 34 weeks. Many staff interpreted this literally to mean that a patient attending for the first time after 28 weeks (which is common in Malawi) should not be given any dose at all, since she has missed her first dose, and therefore could not be given a 'second' dose. Interviews with women showed that less than half knew why they should be taking SP in pregnancy, and so many refused; women who understood why PIT was important were more likely to comply.

The evaluation report was circulated to the District Health Office and partner stakeholders and recommendations were made about how to revise the policy. Since the policy revision would take several months to years, it was also decided to feed back the results of the evaluation to each antenatal clinic in the district. During the evaluation feedback, the policy and guidelines were simplified and discussed with antenatal clinic staff. Clinic patient flow and staff

> **Box 14.2 Case study. Feeding back results to antenatal clinic staff and patients in Malawi** *(cont)*
>
> procedures were reorganized to facilitate directly observed treatment. Staff were shown the position of their clinic in a 'blind' league table to motivate their compliance with the new procedures. Posters were made for women to explain the need to take SP during pregnancy.
>
> A follow-up evaluation showed an increase in the proportion of women receiving at least two doses of PIT-SP (from 48 to 69%) in line with the Abuja target of 60%. There were improvements in the timing of doses and the practice of directly observed treatment.

antenatal visit) and HIV-infected women. Thus, in feeding back to clients and antenatal service providers quickly deaths were averted in the district.

Summary

The need to feed back faster to those involved in research and evaluation is now being recognized; key public health agencies are more readily producing practitioner resources for health professionals involved in decision-making stimulated by the belief that policy and practice decisions should be informed by syntheses of research evidence (Armstrong *et al.* 2007). What is also needed are support mechanisms to help stakeholder participants, especially practitioners, to not only implement policy and guidelines but to be responsive to short-term changes as suggested by mid-term evaluations or interim research reports. There needs to be a balance between waiting for a conclusive evidence base and subsequent policy, and making appropriate changes to health promotion practice on the basis of the results of local evaluations and research.

Key points

♦ Most feedback from evaluation is 'upwards' to stakeholder decision-makers.

♦ The time lag between getting research and evaluation results and changing policy and practice is too long.

♦ This time lag is due to an over-emphasis on internal validity in controlled situations rather than the external validity of interventions in everyday contexts.

♦ Feeding back results to stakeholder participants is important to fulfill ethical obligations; to provide an opportunity to learn and alter the intervention and inform external validity.

♦ Health promotion as a discipline needs to strike a balance between the time taken to produce a strong evidence base and the immediate needs of practitioners and users.

References

Armstrong, R., Waters, E., Crockett, B., and Keleher, H. (2007) The nature of evidence resources and knowledge translation for health promotion practitioners. *Health Promotion International* **22**(3), 254–63.

Ashwood-Smith, H., Coombes, Y., Kaimila, N., Bokosi, M., and Lungu, K. (2002) Availability and use of sulphadoxine-pyrimethamine and iron in pregnancy in Blantyre District. *Malawi Medical Journal* **14**(1), 8–11.

Balas, E.A. and Boren, S.A. (2000) Managing clinical knowledge for health care improvement. In J. Bemmel and A.T. McCray, eds, *Yearbook of Medical Informatics*, pp. 65–70. Schattauer Publishing, Stuttgart.

Beauchamp, T.L. and Childress, J.F. (1989) *Principles of Biomedical Ethics*. Oxford University Press, Oxford.

Bero, L.A., Grilli, R., Grimshaw, J.M., Harvey, E., Oxman, A.D., and Thomson, M. (1998) Closing the gap between research and practice: an overview of systematic reviews of interventions to promote the implementation of research findings. *British Medical Journal* **317**, 465–8.

Brownson, R.C., Ballew, P., Brown, K.L., Elliott, M., Haire-Joshu, D., Heath, G.W., and Kreuter, M.W. (2007) The effect of disseminating evidence-based interventions that promote physical activity to health departments. *American Journal of Public Health* **97**(10), 1900–7.

Coombes, Y., Ashwood-Smith, H., Kaimila, N., Campbell, C.H., Bokosi, M., Mwalwanda, E., and Lungu, K. (2003) *Achieving the Abuja Target for Preventive Intermittent Treatment for Malaria in Pregnancy using a Tailored Feedback Intervention in Blantyre District, Malawi*. Report for Blantyre Integrated Malaria Initiative.

Glasgow, R.E., Lichtenstein, E., and Marcus, A.C. (2003) Why don't we see more translation of health promotion research to practice? Rethinking the efficacy to effectiveness transition. *American Journal of Public Health* **93**(8), 1261–8.

Green, L. and Mercer, S. (2001) Can public health researchers and agencies reconcile the push from funding bodies and the pull from communities? *American Journal of Public Health* **91**(12), 1926–9.

Marie Stopes International (2007) *Social Franchising Project for Modern Clinical Family Planning Methods. End of Project Evaluation Report*. Marie Stopes International, London.

Steckler, A. and McLeroy, K. (2008) The importance of external validity. *American Journal of Public Health* **98**(1), 9–10.

WHO/UNAIDS (2007) *Technical Consultation Male Circumcision and HIV Prevention: Research Implications for Policy and Programming*. Montreux, 6–8 March 2007.

Chapter 15

Getting findings into policy

Carol Tannahill

One criterion against which to measure the success of an evaluation is whether it is of use. This chapter focuses on the usefulness of findings for policy-makers. It starts by looking briefly at the concept of evidence-based policy-making and then reviews some of the ways in which policy might be influenced by research ideas and findings, illustrating these processes with an example from Scotland.

Evidence and policy

A key feature of the modern policy-making process (Cabinet Office 1999) is that policy should be evidence-based. Other features include the need to be forward- and outward-looking, innovative, flexible, and creative, and to take a holistic view. Policy should also be regularly and systematically reviewed.

There are many resources and networks in place in the UK to support links between evidence and policy (for example, the policy hub at <http://www.nationalschool.gov.uk/policyhub/> and the Evidence for Policy and Practice Information and Coordinating (EPPI) Centre at <http://eppi.ioe.ac.uk/cms/>). The arguments are that resources should be focused on what works and on reaching those with greatest need, that policy should avoid doing harm or reinventing the wheel, and that there is value in incorporating learning about implementation processes.

There is, however, a substantial critique of the drive towards evidence-based policy that urges the need for caution concerning evaluations and their conclusions. At its simplest, the argument is that a process evaluation will tell you *how* intervention X worked in Y circumstances. An impact (or outcome) evaluation will tell you that intervention A resulted in B outcomes for people of type C in D circumstances. Rarely will a single evaluation provide a sufficient basis for policy development. Evidence synthesis, from a range of sources and incorporating different types of evidence, will help (see Chapter 3), and evaluators should ensure that their work is written up in a way that enables their findings to be synthesized with others (see Chapter 6). However, even review-level evidence (often regarded as the pinnacle of the evidence hierarchy) has limitations as a basis for predicting the effects of policies, and will not always be the most useful or appropriate (Petticrew and Roberts 2003).

Robson (2002) reminds us that it is 'open systems' (those in which not all aspects can be controlled) that are predominant in society and this has implications for research and its interpretation (see Chapter 10 on natural experiments).

> In closed systems, explanation and prediction are symmetrical; if we can explain, we can predict, and vice versa. But in open systems, the actual configurations of structures and processes are constantly changing, making definite prediction impossible.
>
> (Robson 2002, p. 41)

Policy-makers are alert to the impossibility of predicting exact effects, but need to take decisions based on the best possible knowledge. In England the National Institute for Health and Clinical Excellence (NICE) is central to the knowledge-transfer process (see Chapter 12). In creating a framework for public health guidance, Kelly and colleagues argue that whereas 'individual difference and variability is the stuff of human life', which makes prediction hard at the level of individual behaviour, the patterning of experience at group and population levels does enable accurate aggregate predictions to be drawn (Kelly *et al.* 2008). Four vectors of causation—population, environmental, organizational, and social—are instrumental in creating these patterns. It follows that health promotion evaluations should include attention to these vectors as well as to the specific intervention or policy of interest.

Tannahill (2008) makes the case for further emphasizing *good decision-making* as an objective. Evidence is an insufficient basis for that. Instead he proposes a health-improvement 'decision-making triangle' which gives primacy to a set of ethical principles, with evidence and theory informing their application. If such an approach were more widely adopted, the challenge for health promotion evaluation would be to consider more systematically how the evaluation might shed light on principles such as sustainability, social responsibility, equity, and accountability.

The routes from research to policy

The experience of evaluators over time has shown that there is no simple, linear route leading from the publication of findings to their integration into policy. Early analyses focused on dissemination as the primary activity, with useful insights such as those of Crossthwaite and Curtice (1994) helping in differentiating different models (see Box 15.1). The rational model is recognized as the least effective: the insider model as having the potential to maximize research relevance, utilization and influence.

An analysis (Smith 2008) of the relationship between research on health inequalities in the UK and the policy responses which emerged in Scotland and England found little evidence that policies were based on evidence but much to support the thesis that research-based *ideas* had travelled into policy. Ideas that posed no challenge to institutionalized beliefs or that could be transformed into more flexible, less-demanding

---

Box 15.1 Four models of dissemination of research to policy-makers

The rational model	By making information available it will be used to inform policy-making.
The lime-stone model	The relationship is less direct, with research findings trickling in a slower and less predictable way into policy.
The gadfly model	Dissemination is planned and given a lot of attention, ensuring feedback meetings to different stakeholders, use of media, etc.
The insider model	Researchers have direct links with policy-makers. (Crossthwaite and Curtice 1994)

prospects were more 'successful' at making their way into policy than those that would be more transformative and challenging to prevailing institutions and understandings.

More generally, attention has moved away from dissemination towards knowledge transfer and, more ambitiously, knowledge use. This requires researchers to think about the characteristics, situations, and requirements of those they want to respond to their findings. Users are regarded as active participants in the process, not passive receivers. For Nutley *et al.* (2002), knowledge use 'has been reconceptualized as a learning process, in which new knowledge is shaped by the learner's pre-existing knowledge and experience.' Findings will be dealt with differently depending on the policy-maker's interests, knowledge, experience, and circumstance. At a minimum, the researcher needs to be alert to this.

Taking these ideas a stage further, the likelihood of research influencing policy is increased when policy-makers have a role not only in responding to findings, but also in shaping the research. This can happen even in a researcher-led approach (as opposed to the well-established 'commissioned research' mode), through processes of stakeholder consultation and involvement. Benefits of co-creation are well established in a range of arenas (from product development to organizational learning) and can be realized in research without compromising the integrity of the academic process.

Dissemination, the influence of ideas, knowledge use, and co-creation are not mutually exclusive processes. The influence of research on policy still happens in slightly mysterious ways, but attention to building the narrative and ideas from your research, and learning about and working with those you want to influence with your findings, will be time well spent.

Competing priorities and practical considerations

The principle of bridging the gap between research and policy is one that is readily accepted, but its delivery involves reconciling differences and confronting some practical considerations. Although things are changing, incentives and opportunities for researchers still primarily lie in traditional academic research. Career progression depends on peer review, publication, and grant income; communication skills are those required for an academic audience; valued knowledge is primarily technical and specialist; ownership of ideas and data are closely guarded to protect intellectual property; and timescales are long (the many months it can take for a journal article to be published is one example).

Contrast this with the policy-making world, where timescales are driven by political terms (usually 3 or 4 years); language has to be non-technical; academic journals are not the primary source of information; and public opinion is the major influence. To influence policy, the research process needs to find a 'fit' with this world as well as with that of academia. Sometimes a single process and set of products will fulfil both sets of requirements: more often academic dissemination and policy influence involve different (concurrent or sequential) processes.

A third dimension also needs consideration: that of the research sponsor, or funder. Evaluation findings not uncommonly are challenging to those who have funded the evaluations (often the funder is the service provider or commissioner, or has some particular interest in the intervention being studied). Researchers may find themselves being asked to revise findings or recommendations, or not to make them public, in order to alleviate sponsors' concerns about how they are portrayed. Clear agreements should be reached at the start of the evaluation process on how such circumstances will be managed should they arise.

Finally, despite every best effort, the reality is that the change process is generally more complex than anticipated. It almost always involves a tug of war between the principle of remaining true to the evidence on the one hand and the pragmatism of doing what is feasible and acceptable on the other.

Influencing policy: an example

All of these issues are evident in the following case study describing GoWell, the Glasgow Community Health and Wellbeing Research and Learning Programme.

Case study: GoWell

GoWell is a long-term study exploring the processes of neighbour-hood regeneration and their impacts on the health and wellbeing of individuals and communities in 14 areas of Glasgow. Regeneration policy is developed nationally in Scotland and also locally in Glasgow. It seeks to be holistic, to draw on evidence from across disciplines, and to impact on many dimensions of people's lives. Key outcomes of interest for GoWell relate to housing, the environment, community cohesion and empowerment, and health and wellbeing. Very little is known about the impacts of area-based regeneration programmes on health (Thomson *et al.* 2006) but there is a predominant idea (which has made its way into policy) that regeneration is a route to better health (see Chapter 6 for a description of a systematic review of housing regeneration and health). There is therefore a need to build the evidence base in a way that tests that idea.

The study involves a mix of qualitative and quantitative methods, and primary and secondary research. Each component aims to answer a different set of questions, in line with the approach proposed by Petticrew and Roberts (2003). The range of study areas, and their location within a wider process of ecological monitoring, enables some assessment of the transferability of findings.

GoWell is a partnership between the Glasgow Centre for Population Health, the University of Glasgow, and the MRC Social and Public Health Sciences Unit. The team is multi-disciplinary in nature, with researchers at its core, to ensure that the research is high quality and can support the programme's other aims (including policy influence). But other team members bring skills in communication, policy development, and programme implementation and management.

The programme is sponsored by:

+ Glasgow Housing Association (landlord to many of the participants, and a primary deliverer of the interventions of interest);

+ Scottish Government (whose policies are driving much of the change);

+ NHS Health Scotland (the national health-improvement organization); and

♦ NHS Greater Glasgow and Clyde (the local Health Board/ Authority).

All sponsors and partners sit on the programme steering group (enabling the insider model and a degree of co-creation), alongside three external academic advisors (who review and advise on the research methodology). There have been difficult issues when findings have been challenging to one of the sponsors, but no individual organization can veto publication. Dissemination and communication strategies were agreed by the steering group at the outset and are reviewed regularly.

Four years into the study there are regular (at least six per annum) seminars and discussion meetings with policy-makers within Glasgow and nationally. Together the researchers and policy-makers work to distil recommendations and policy implications from the research findings. Local tenants and residents have also begun to use the findings, and are requesting analyses of interest to them. It appears that most of the pieces of the jigsaw are in place for GoWell's findings to find their way into policy in the future, and that is the expectation of Scottish politicians and civil servants, but time will tell. More information on GoWell can be found at <http://www.gowellonline.co.uk>.

Conclusion

There are many reasons for evaluators to be concerned with getting their findings into policy. Research commissioners are placing increasing emphasis on the impact achieved from the research they have funded, with researchers being asked to provide evidence of this 'added value'. But even without this contractual expectation, researchers generally want to ensure that their research 'does good'. Policy influence is one of the primary routes to achieving this.

Just as a concern with evaluation should be built into any policy or intervention from the start, so should early attention be paid to the purpose of the evaluation (see Chapter 3). In order to get findings into policy, evaluators need to be concerned not only with academic rigour (including the quality of the methodology and robustness of the results) but also with issues of policy relevance, timeliness, transferability of findings, and implications for implementation. Skills in research communication and dissemination, and an ability to put findings into context are essential. There is much more to influencing policy than 'simply' doing a good evaluation. Evaluators must learn new skills in communicating their findings to policy-makers and in working with the timescales and priorities of policy-makers.

Key points

- Policy-makers are one group for whom health promotion evaluation should be useful. Good policy-making should take account of evidence as one of its guiding principles.

- Evidence can also contribute to other policy-making principles (such as being outward-looking, taking a holistic view, and being inclusive).

- This has implications for the types of evidence needed to inform policy. The traditional evidence hierarchy will not always be appropriate. The concepts of open systems, vectors of causation, and ethical decision-making are useful developments with implications for evaluation design.

- Doing good-quality evaluation is only the first step towards getting findings into policy. Researchers also need to pay attention to building the narrative and ideas that flow from the findings, and to learning and acknowledging policy-makers' interests, experience, and aspirations.

- Researchers, funders, and policy-makers work to different timescales and priorities. Finding a way to manage these conflicting requirements, without compromising the integrity of the research process, is essential if researchers want to influence policy.

References

Cabinet Office (1999) *Professional Policy Making for the Twenty First Century*. <http://www.nationalschool.gov.uk/policyhub/docs/profpolicymaking.pdf>. Cabinet Office, London.

Crossthwaite, C. and Curtice, L. (1994) Disseminating research results – the challenge of bridging the gap between health research and health action. *Health Promotion International* **9**(4), 289–96.

Kelly, M.P., Stewart, E., Morgan, A. et al. (2008) A conceptual framework for public health: NICE's emerging approach. *Public Health* **123**, e14–20.

Nutley, S., Walter, I., and Davies, H.T.O. (2002) *From Knowing to Doing: A Framework for Understanding the Evidence-into-Practice Agenda.* Discussion Paper 1, Research Unit for Research Utilisation, University of St Andrews, St Andrews.

Petticrew, M. and Roberts, H. (2003) Evidence, hierarchies, and typologies: horses for courses. *Journal of Epidemiology and Community Health* **57**, 527–9.

Robson, C. (2002) *Real World Research: A Resource for Social Scientists and Practitioner-Researchers*, 2nd edn. Blackwell Publishing, Oxford.

Smith, K.E. (2008) *Health Inequalities in Scotland and England: the Translation of Ideas Between Research and Policy.* PhD thesis, University of Edinburgh.

Tannahill, A. (2008) Beyond evidence – to ethics: a decision-making framework for health promotion, public health and health improvement. *Health Promotion International* **23**(4), 380–90.

Thomson, H., Atkinson, R., Petticrew, M., and Kearns, A. (2006) Do urban regeneration programmes improve public health and reduce health inequalities? A synthesis of the evidence from UK policy and practice (1980–2004). *Journal of Epidemiology & Community Health* **60**, 108–15.

Chapter 16

Conclusions: providing appropriate evidence and influencing policy

Margaret Thorogood and
Yolande Coombes

We hope that this book has provided a panoramic view of how health promotion can and should be evaluated, not forgetting that the primary reason for any evaluation is to inform and influence decisions, whether of health practitioners, funders or policy-makers. The twenty-first century has seen health promotion come of age, no longer described as a fuzzy concept, and now with a coherent approach and a clear mandate. As health promotion has achieved maturity so the methods by which health promotion and public health are evaluated have evolved. In contrast to the situation when the last edition of this book was published, there is no longer a debate about the relative value of quantitative and qualitative research methods. Mixed-methods approaches to evaluation are now widely accepted and are constantly being developed and refined. Discussion now centres around how and when the two methods should be combined. Reflecting this situation, almost all of the chapters in this book describe the use of some combination of quantitative and qualitative methods. While peace has broken out in the methodology wars with the acceptance of a mixed-methods approach, many tensions remain in health promotion evaluations.

Internal versus external validity: a creative tension

Although some of the debates in health promotion evaluations may be resolved in time, others should be regarded as permanent sources of a creative tension that will need to be addressed and resolved freshly in each new evaluation. One of the most important of these creative tensions is that between using a rigorous research design to achieve internal validity and adapting an intervention to circumstances in ways which enhance external validity. This issue has been visited throughout the book. In Part II, on methods of evaluation, this issue is discussed in most of the chapters. Chapter 3 discusses the important need for evaluations which provide evidence in real-world settings (having strong external validity) and how this involves examining process, inputs, and outcomes. In Chapter 4 Britton reviews how both internal and external validity can be strengthened or compromised according to how experimental evaluations are designed. In Chapter 5, on economic evaluation, Stevens calls for greater transparency in the reporting of both methods and results to enable interpretations of both internal and external validity. Ellard and Parsons describe in Chapter 7 how process evaluation can illuminate the external validity of an intervention. The tensions between internal and external validity are also touched on in others chapters, such as Chapter 10 on environmental interventions, Chapter 11 on e-health, and Chapter 9 on intimate partner violence.

A dichotomy may appear to exist between whether an evaluation should focus on achieving internal or external validity, but the ideal approach is more complex. There is not a simple choice with one right answer, but rather that there is a correct approach, which is to be aware of this tension and manage it in the way that is appropriate to the purpose of the evaluation being carried out. It is important to provide evidence for both the efficacy and effectiveness of health promotion interventions. In some instances it is possible to do this with one study or evaluation; but in most cases evidence must be pieced together from many different evaluations that take different approaches using a mixture of methods.

Coping with the complexity and designing appropriate evaluations

Another theme that runs through this book is the complex nature of many health promotion interventions, which in turn stems from the complex nature of health and of the factors that affect health. In our introduction we discussed the four vectors of health (population, environmental, organizational, and social) and the social ecological approach which looks at determinants of health at every level (from individual, through family, community, to society and even globally). In Chapter 10 Hillsdon also points out that the determinants of health impact at many different levels from the macroeconomy to individual behaviour change and that health promotion can work at all these levels. Coombes discusses in Chapter 3 the problem of health promotion interventions failing to concentrate on a holistic model of health but rather focusing on physical health gain to the detriment of social, economic, or emotional health gain, and in Chapter 2 Berridge shows how the focus on different determinants of health has shifted over time and with different policy emphasis.

Linked to the complexity of health promotion interventions is the necessity of designing studies that are appropriate to the purpose of the evaluation. Evaluations can range from simple, inexpensive audits of activity to large, complex, and very expensive, randomized controlled trials. In Chapter 6 Thorogood reminds us that systematic reviews have an important role to play in assembling and evaluating the evidence of effectiveness in health promotion; a role that is not limited to quantitative analysis of randomized controlled trials but offers wider opportunities to understand findings and identify research gaps. It is important to fit the evaluation to the purpose. As Coombes has argued, evidence should be regarded as lying on a continuum from evidence of efficacy (which is often derived from randomized trials and can be very expensive to collect) to evidence, for example, of levels of uptake in the population (counting heads) of an already proven effective intervention being introduced to a new setting. She calls for evaluation programmes to be designed in a way that is appropriate to the decisions that will be made on the basis of the evaluation. Similarly, Ellard and Parsons (Chapter 7) argue that the design of process evaluation studies, like the design of any research study, must be led by the research questions that need to be answered.

Ellard and Parsons go on to review how an understanding of the process of an intervention is crucial to interpreting the complexity of an intervention and its external and internal validity. As they argue, there is an increasing need to carry out process evaluations alongside studies of effectiveness. External effectiveness is not only determined by the content of the intervention but also by the way that it is implemented and by the experiences, beliefs, and attitudes of the people that participate.

Both Chapter 8 on social marketing and Chapter 9 on intimate partner violence demonstrate how using inappropriate methodologies to understand complex interventions lead to spurious results which are of no value. In Chapter 8 Chapman describes how social marketing interventions should be assessed against six benchmark criteria which should be universally adopted. Without these criteria, activities which are not social marketing are evaluated inappropriately, and others which are social marketing are ignored. Jewkes in Chapter 9 reminds us that for interventions on intimate partner violence change often occurs over long time frames, so evaluations need to be appropriately designed; she also comments on the fact that interventions must be shown to have been adequately developed and their potential understood before a major evaluation is attempted.

Chapters 10 on environmental changes and Chapter 11 on e-health promotion show how the complexity of an intervention can be incorporated into a study design. Hillsdon (Chapter 10) describes how natural experiments in the built environment provide an opportunity to evaluate the effectiveness of interventions when complex randomized controlled trials are not feasible. In discussing the opportunities for e-health promotion, Powell explains how the broad methodological approaches recommended for use in e-health promotion are the same as for health promotion in general, but e-health evaluation presents new opportunities and challenges, such as the ability to conduct whole trials online, and to collect new process measures.

Feeding into policy

One of the important aims of any evaluation is to inform decision-making, by either the funders of the intervention or, on a wider scale, the makers of health-related policy. In the past there has been a tendency to assume that once policy-makers are given the scientific evidence then it will be translated into policy. Even the most superficial study of the relationship between policy and evidence will show that this is sadly not the case. There is an increasing awareness that if an evaluation is to have any influence then the researchers undertaking the evaluation must be proactive in bringing this about. Most people undertaking health promotion evaluation will feel that there is no point in undertaking the evaluation unless the results are going to influence policy, yet often neglect to take any steps to make their finding influence policy. In Chapter 15, Tannahill describes how she and her team have designed an evaluation which involves the policy-makers right from the start and aims to feed directly into decision-making. Coombes in Chapter 14 reminds us that it is also important to feedback findings to the people who participated in the study, as a courtesy certainly, but more importantly to give them the information they need to become more effective in what they are trying to do. Cowl, in Chapter 12, writing from the perspective of the policy-maker, turns the argument round and talks about the equally important issue of how to involve the lay public (ordinary people) in developing policy.

In the conclusion to the last edition of this book we wrote:

> We did not intend that this book would comprise a complete enumeration of all the available methods for evaluating health promotion. Indeed, we doubt that any definitive list of such methods could be drawn up, since new approaches are constantly being developed. However, we have aimed to include a wide spectrum of examples from diverse cultural and economic contexts and to include some of the most topical and important issues in health promotion evaluation.

(Thorogood and Coombes 2004, p. 177)

In this edition we have included some of these new approaches (for example, the evaluation of e-health and natural experiments, and involving lay people in the policy process). We aimed to provide content that reflects some of the current issues in health promotion, most notably how to strengthen the health promotion evidence base, and how to maximize internal and external validity. We have provided examples of different approaches to evaluating what are, almost always, complex interventions for health promotion. But our final plea is the need to integrate evaluation more firmly into the policy process. It took more than 30 years for the evidence on smoking and its effects on health to be translated into national policy, and nearer half a century before effective strategy such as banning smoking in workplaces emerged. There is a temptation to want to constantly improve evaluation methodology, building an ever-more watertight case for an intervention, while ignoring the need for action. If our work in evaluating health promotion is to contribute effectively to better health then it must be translated into policy. To do this, researchers must engage with those who make decisions and shape policy, by providing and interpreting the evidence they need. A theme of this book has been that evaluations should be designed to answer predetermined appropriate questions. The most effective evaluations will be those that engage decision-makers from the start in determining the questions. In addition, effective researchers must ensure that results are not buried in academic journals but are fed back to participants, to funders, to the wider health economy, and to those who shape policy.

Key points

- Health promotion evaluation requires the use of mixed methods.
- It is often not possible to achieve internal and external validity in the same piece of research, so evidence should be built incrementally.
- Health promotion interventions are complex and evaluations must take account of this complexity.
- Evaluation is only valuable if it informs decisions.
- Researchers should engage actively with participants, funders, the wider health economy, and those who shape policy.

Reference

Thorogood, M. and Coombes, Y. (2004) Conclusions: integrating methods for practice. In M. Thorogood and Y. Coombes, eds, *Evaluating Health Promotion: Practice and Methods*, 2nd edn, pp. 177–81. Oxford University Press, Oxford.

Index

Note: Page references to tables are in *italics* and those to figures are in **bold**.